Older Lesbian, Gay, Bisexual and Trans People

T0179036

What does it mean to grow older as a lesbian, gay, bisexual or trans (LGBT) person? What gaps in knowledge about LGBT ageing remain? This timely and innovative book reports on a project funded by the Economic and Social Research Council which aimed to address gaps in knowledge about older LGBT people and their experiences of ageing. The book discusses the project and contains chapters either specially commissioned or written by leading researchers and activists in the field.

Informed by a range of theoretical perspectives, empirical research studies, critical observations, as well as lived experiences, this book explores areas of LGBT ageing that have been under-studied. These include: bisexual ageing; trans ageing and older trans people's mental health; ethnicity, culture and religion in the lives of older LGBT people and gaps in knowledge about older LGBT people from minority ethnic communities; intergenerational networks; residential and end-of-life care; and the effects of austerity on services.

Written in an accessible style, this book is essential for researchers and policy makers interested in the lives of older LGBT people, people who work with older people, and teachers and students interested in ageing, gender identity and sexuality.

Andrew King is Professor of Sociology at the University of Surrey, UK, where he also co-directs the Centre for Research on Ageing and Gender (CRAG). He has researched and written about LGBT ageing for more than ten years.

Kathryn Almack is Professor of Health, Young People and Family Lives in Health and Social Work at the University of Hertfordshire. She has researched and written on LGBT family lives across the life course over the past twenty years, with a focus on LGBT end-of-life care over the past ten years.

Yiu-tung Suen is Assistant Professor on the Gender Studies Programme at the Chinese University of Hong Kong. He is the Founding Director of the Sexualities Research Programme, the first research programme in Hong Kong dedicated to conducting rigorous, independent research on sexuality issues, with a focus on sexual orientation, gender identity, law and social policy.

Sue Westwood is a freelance researcher and writer, and an Associate Lecturer with the Open University. She has published widely in the field of LGBT ageing.

Older Lesbian, Gay, Bisexual and Trans People

Minding the Knowledge Gaps

**Edited by Andrew King, Kathryn Almack,
Yiu-Tung Suen and Sue Westwood**

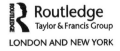

Routledge
Taylor & Francis Group

LONDON AND NEW YORK

First published 2019
by Routledge
2 Park Square, Milton Park, Abingdon, Oxon OX14 4RN

and by Routledge
52 Vanderbilt Avenue, New York, NY 10017, USA

First issued in paperback 2020

Routledge is an imprint of the Taylor & Francis Group, an informa business

British Library Cataloguing-in-Publication Data
A catalogue record for this book is available from the British Library

Library of Congress Cataloging-in-Publication Data
Names: King, Andrew, editor. | Almack, Kathryn, editor. | Suen, Yiu Tung, editor.
Title: Older lesbian, gay, bisexual and trans people : minding the knowledge gaps / edited by Andrew King, Kathryn Almack, Yiu-tung Suen.
Description: New York : Routledge, 2018. | Series: Routledge advances in social work | Includes bibliographical references and index.
Identifiers: LCCN 2018019295 | ISBN 9781138644939 (hardback) | ISBN 9781315628462 (ebook)
Subjects: LCSH: Older sexual minorities—Social conditions. | Aging. | Sexual minorities—Services for.
Classification: LCC HQ73 .O43 2018 | DDC 306.76084/6—dc23
LC record available at https://lccn.loc.gov/2018019295

ISBN 13: 978-0-367-58608-9 (pbk)
ISBN 13: 978-1-138-64493-9 (hbk)

Typeset in Times New Roman
by codeMantra

Contents

Illustrations

Figure

Tables

Foreword

The year 2017 saw the widely celebrated fiftieth anniversary of the passing of the 1967 Sexual Offences Act. This legislated the partial decriminalisation of male homosexuality, for those aged over 21, in private, as long as one lived in England and Wales, and did not serve in the armed services or merchant navy. As this suggests, it was a severely limited piece of legislation. It did not refer to women, let alone bisexuals or trans people, did not apply to Scotland and Northern Ireland until the early 1980s, and involved a very narrow definition of privacy. It was to take nearly 40 years more before full legal equality was achieved in the early 2000s. The significance of this slice of history is that those LGBT+ people now moving into older age have lived most of their lives in conditions of illegality, inequality, invisibility, silence, discrimination and prejudice.

Much has changed for the better since 1967, largely as a result of the activities of LGBT+ people themselves. But as the contributors to this book powerfully remind us, the scars of those years still shape the consciousness, fears and life experiences, as well as the hopes and desires, of older LGBT+ people. And societal responses to the needs of older LGBT+ people are, consciously or unconsciously, still marked by that history. An inequitable (and iniquitous) past, as Andrew King points out in his chapter in this book, continues to limit the achievement of full and equal citizenship in the present and for the future.

The LGBT+ world is not a single homogeneous entity. It is multifarious, multivocal and hugely diverse, with different experiences and needs. Links between people are not laid down by nature; they have to be (often painfully) constructed, and nourished. Bi and trans people have often found it difficult to make their voices heard and their particular struggles recognised. While younger people can readily accept gender and sexual fluidity, older LGBT+ people often have a strong sense of their identities which have been struggled for over many years. These very identities have different meanings and implications if one is from a BAME community and marked by the experience of racism both outside and within the LGBT+ world. Above all, age remains a major determinant of difference and potential division, intersecting with all the other vectors of power and discrimination.

We are shaped by our generation, as various contributors demonstrate. Generational differences embody different life experiences, and different perspectives on the world. As the sociologist Ken Plummer has observed, there are 'generational sexualities', through which attitudes and beliefs derived from changing social worlds give rise to different stories about the past and present. Crucially, different generations of the same chronological age group can coexist, side by side. Any group of older LGBT+ people can contain several different sexual and gender generations: lesbian and gay men who experienced the liberatory politics of the 1970s and changed their lives radically alongside men and women who have come out for the first time in old age; bi and trans activists who struggled to affirm their sense of self in long periods of isolation or enforced privacy, alongside the newer, more assertive expressions of sexual and gender fluidity today.

Just as a sense of generational belonging is complex and challenging, so is a sense of time. Ruth Pearce's contribution to the book speaks of 'trans-time', which is non-linear, related not to chronological age but to social experience, and in particular to the anticipations of transition. More broadly, the idea of queer time has been used to describe the different rhythms and demands marked and made by specific histories of exclusion, oppression and resistance – continuing into our current age if austerity – on the lives of older LGBT+ people.

Older LGBT+ people have rich and varied histories, and different needs and desires, vividly delineated in the various chapters of this book. What they have in common is the right to be heard, to be understood, and to have full and equal access to care, attention and social justice. All that, in turn, requires the right to be known about. This book makes a vital contribution to our knowledge of older LGBT+ people. Without knowledge there can be no justice. And without justice there can be no full citizenship and belonging.

Professor Jeffrey Weeks
May 2018

Acknowledgements

As editors of this book we would like to acknowledge and thank a number of people. First, we would like to thank all those individuals who attended and/or presented at the ESRC-funded seminar series 'Older LGBT People: Minding the Knowledge Gaps' on which this book is based. It was a whirlwind 18 months but very supportive, and it would not have been possible without all those who attended and contributed. Second, we would like to thank Georgia Priestly and all at Routledge for their support in bringing this book to publication.

Andrew King, Kathryn Almack, Yiu-Tung Suen and Sue Westwood

Contributors

Kathryn Almack is Professor of Health and Family Lives in the School of Health and Social Work at the University of Hertfordshire. She is a sociologist whose research addresses family lives, health and well-being across the life course. Over the past decade, her work has had a substantial focus on lesbian, gay, bisexual and trans (LGBT) older people, ageing and end-of-life care. She has completed a number of funded projects and published widely in this area. Findings from her research have been used to develop new resources for practitioners and policy makers. She is co-editor of *Intersections of Ageing, Gender and Sexualities* (with Andrew King and Rebecca Jones) and serves on the editorial board for the British Sociological Association journal *Sociology*. She is currently researching lesbian parenthood as part of a longitudinal qualitative research project.

Louis Bailey is a Research Fellow in Sociology at the University of Hull. His research focuses on trans people's experiences across the life course and in relation to ageing and end of life. He was co-author of the *Trans Mental Health Study* (2012) and has published papers on health and social inequalities, suicide prevention, bereavement and memorialisation. Outside of academia, Louis is an artist and the co-founding director of 'Artmob', a fledgling visual arts organisation promoting the work of trans and non-binary artists. As part of 'Artmob', Louis co-curated the exhibition 'Continuum: Framing Trans Lives in Twenty-First Century Britain' – which featured the work of 14 trans and non-binary artists – at the People's History Museum, Manchester. In his own visual and written practice, Louis explores gender variance as tied to physical and mental endurance both across the socio-political landscape and the shifting natural world. He is currently working on his first collection of creative non-fiction, 'The Night Run'.

Malen Davies a Senior Researcher working across the Social Attitudes and Children, Families and Work teams at NatCen. She is a qualitative specialist and is working on a broad range of research projects. She has recently managed a project for the Equality and Human Right Commission focusing on equality and diversity, which involved developing guidance documents for employers on how to interpret the Equality Act in relation to Religion or Belief. Malen's interests include equality and diversity, the labour market and improving access to good-quality jobs for disadvantaged groups.

Sonja J. Ellis is an Associate Professor in Human Development at the University of Waikato, Aotearoa/New Zealand. Sonja has researched and published widely on issues affecting LGBTIQ people; she is a co-author of the textbook *Lesbian, Gay, Bisexual, Trans and Queer Psychology: An introduction*, published by Cambridge University Press. Sonja was part of the research team for the UK *Trans Mental Health Study*, and has co-published a number of papers from this project with her colleagues Louis Bailey (University of Hull) and Jay McNeil (Independent Researcher). Her current research projects include a collaborative study with Damien Riggs (University of Adelaide) and Gareth Treharne (University of Otago), exploring social connectedness and suicide risk in gender-diverse persons in Australia and New Zealand. She is also undertaking a research project – supervised by Robyn Aitken (Charles Darwin University) – on the sexual health education needs of adolescents in New Zealand.

Sue George is a writer, editor and activist who has identified as bisexual since 1973 and has been in and around the British bisexual community since the mid-1980s. Her book *Women and Bisexuality*, which came out in 1993, was the first (and so far only) book on the subject to be published in the UK. She has also written about bisexuality for many publications and has blogged at BisexualityandBeyond.com since 2006. Her more recent work is focused around the issues of bisexuality and older people, as well as the history of bisexuality. She is currently involved in setting up an oral history project with people involved in the bi community since the 1980s.

Rebecca L. Jones is a Senior Lecturer in Health at The Open University, UK. She researches ageing, sexuality and, especially, sexuality in later life. She has published widely on topics including ageism and age discrimination, imagining personal ageing, older women's talk about sex, bisexuality, LGBT issues in health and social care and LGBT ageing. She is one of the authors of *The Bisexuality Report* and is best known for her work on ageing and bisexuality.

Andrew King is Professor of Sociology in the Department of Sociology, University of Surrey, UK where he is also Co-Director of the Centre for Research on Ageing and Gender (CRAG). Andrew has published widely in the field of LGBT ageing. His monograph, *Older Lesbian, Gay, Bisexual Adults: identities, intersections, institutions* was published by Routledge in 2016. He is co-editor (with Kathryn Almack and Rebecca L. Jones) of *Intersections of Ageing, Gender and Sexualities*, and has published in a wide range of journals. Andrew's research projects cover different aspects of LGBT ageing, including housing and social care. His current project, funded by the Norface consortium of European Research Councils, examines intersectional life course inequalities among LGBTQI+ people and runs from 2018 to 2021.

Dylan Kneale is a Principal Research Fellow at UCL based at the EPPI Centre (Evidence for Policy and Practice Information and Co-ordinating Centre, UCL Institute of Education). Relationships have been a common thread across much of Dylan's research and he has authored publications examining social isolation, social exclusion, LGBT relationships, family formation, family separation, intergenerational relationships and processes of community engagement. Much of his current work is dedicated to examining how evidence from research can improve decision making at a local and national level.

Mehul Kotecha is a Senior Researcher at NatCen. He has led on a number of qualitative studies, including evaluations of back-to-work programmes (e.g. process evaluation of the Support for the Very Long-Term Unemployed Trailblazer programme), research into financial and material circumstances in old age (e.g. exploring the relationship between material deprivation and pensioner poverty, and a study which explored older people's attitudes towards the principle of automatic awards of Pension Credit), and research into education and skills (e.g. a study exploring motivations and barriers to part-time post-16 education). Prior to this, Mehul was a Research Fellow at the Institute of Primary Care and Public Health, based at London South Bank University – where he also received his Doctorate in Sociology.

Tracey Maegusuku-Hewett is Senior Lecturer in Social Work at Swansea University. Tracey has worked within nursing, residential, community, voluntary and statutory sector roles with children and adults in her capacity as a support worker, nurse with people with learning disabilities and latterly as a qualified social worker. Her research interests include LGBT people's well-being, equality and social work practice, and evidence-enriched practice.

Joanne McCarthy works as a Clinical Psychologist in HIV & Sexual Health at Positive East London. She is the lead on the Re:Assure project, which is a dedicated project for migrant women living with HIV and who have experienced traumatic events. She obtained her Doctorate in Clinical Psychology from the University of Lincoln. She has clinical and research interests in issues related to identity, sexuality and neuropsychological aspects of HIV, and completed her Doctorate research on Identity Formation and Conflict in older Irish gay men.

Catherine McNamara is a Reader in Applied Theatre, and the Director of Learning, Teaching and Student Experience at The Royal Central School of Speech and Drama (University of London). Recent publications include: 'Methods and Approaches for Working with Trans and/ or

Non-binary Young People in the UK', in *The Handbook of Youth Work Practice*, ed. Pam Alldred, Fiona Cullen et al. (London: Sage, 2018) and a co-edited themed issue of 'Research in Drama Education: The Journal of Applied Theatre and Performance' (the Gender and Sexuality issue) Issue 2 (2013) published by Taylor & Francis (with Dr Stephen Farrier).

Jay McNeil is a Clinical Psychologist and an independent researcher. He was lead researcher of the *Trans Mental Health Study* (2012; recipient of the GIRES Research Award) and has published a number of papers on the health and well-being of trans and non-binary people, particularly in relation to experiences of stigma, discrimination, exclusion, minority stress, health services and institutional power structures. He was Co-Founder of 'Trans Bare All', a voluntary organisation dedicated to the health and well-being of trans people, with a particular focus on body positivity and community empowerment. Jay regularly provides health consultancy and training on gender diversity.

Martin Mitchell is a Research Director within the Social Attitudes team at NatCen. He has worked on a large number of qualitative studies involving the use of in-depth interviews, face-to-face and online focus groups, observations and deliberative methods. He has conducted research in many areas, including equalities and discrimination, bullying and harassment, same-sex relationships, sexual orientation, gender identity, religion and belief, and perceptions of fairness. This has included work funded by the Government Equalities Office, Equality and Human Rights Commission, Acas and the Health & Safety Executive.

Roshan das Nair is Professor of Clinical Psychology & Neuropsychology at the Institute of Mental Health, University of Nottingham. He is a British Psychological Society (BPS) Chartered Clinical Psychologist and a Health and Care Professions' Council Registered Practitioner Psychologist. After completing his clinical training from the National Institute of Mental Health and Neurosciences in India, he obtained his Ph.D. from the University of Nottingham. He previously worked as a Lecturer at the University of Zambia, and until recently he was a Consultant Clinical Psychologist with Nottingham University Hospitals NHS Trust. He was former Editor of the *Psychology of Sexualities Review* (published by the BPS), and has co-edited the book *Intersectionality, Sexuality and Psychological Therapies: Working with lesbian, gay and bisexual diversity* (Wiley, 2012).

Ruth Pearce is a Research Fellow in the School of Sociology and Social Policy at the University of Leeds, UK. Her work explores issues of inequality, marginalisation, power and political struggle from a trans feminist perspective. At the time of writing, she is working as part of an international research team to explore transmasculine people's experiences of pregnancy and childbirth. Ruth's monograph, *Understanding Trans*

Health: Discourse, power and possibility, was published by Policy Press in 2018. She blogs about her work at http://ruthpearce.net.

Michele Raithby is Associate Professor in Social Work at Swansea University. Following work in a variety of research and care settings, Michele qualified in social work at the University of Oxford. Her qualified practice experience includes generic neighbourhood-based social work, specialist mental health social work and inspection of adult residential care services. Her research interests include care and support with older people, and working with gender and sexual diversity in adult social care.

Vernal Scott is an equality and diversity professional, author and ex-man of faith. He is a zestful keynote speaker, media commentator, and facilitator of workshops dealing with the issues raised in his non-fiction book, *God's Other Children: A London memoir*. He also provides confidential support to public and private individuals dealing with sexuality, 'coming out' and sexual health issues, including HIV. Vernal has made impressive contributions to the public and voluntary sector over the past 30 years. In the mid-1980s he launched the 'People's (multi-cultural) Group' at the London Lesbian & Gay Centre, and later founded the 'Black Communities AIDS Team'. In 1987 he was appointed Head of HIV services for Brent, and in 2003 he was appointed Head of Equality and Diversity for Islington, and in 2017 he took up a similar role at Havering, where he works today.

Yiu-Tung Suen is Assistant Professor and Graduate Division Head of the Gender Studies Programme, and Associate Director of the Gender Research Centre, at the Chinese University of Hong Kong. He is Founding Director of the Sexualities Research Programme, the first research programme in Hong Kong dedicated to conducting rigorous, independent research on sexuality issues, with a focus on sexual orientation, gender identity, law and social policy. Internationally, he serves as a consultant and data analyst for the United Nations Development Programme Being LGBTI in Asia Programme, working closely with their Bangkok and Beijing offices. His academic writings may be found published or forthcoming in such journals as *Journal of Homosexuality, Hong Kong Law Journal, Sociological Research Online, Sexual and Relationship Therapy, Higher Education Research and Development, Social Theory and Health*, and others.

Sue Westwood is a freelance researcher and writer, and an Associate Lecturer with The Open University. Her first book, *Ageing, Gender and Sexuality: Equality in later life*, was published by Routledge in 2016 and won the Socio Legal Studies Association (SLSA) Early Career Book Prize for 2017. Her second book, co-edited with Dr Elizabeth Price, *Lesbian, Gay, Bisexual and Trans* (LGBT*) Individuals Living with Dementia: Concepts, practice and rights*, was also published by Routledge in 2016. Her third book, also an edited collection, *Ageing, Diversity and Equality: Social justice perspectives*, was published by Routledge in 2018.

Paul Willis is Senior Lecturer in Social Work in the School for Policy Studies at the University of Bristol. Paul qualified in social work at the University of Tasmania (Australia), and currently teaches community practice and social work with adults on the MSc Social Work Programme at Bristol. His research interests include loneliness and social isolation experienced by older men; sexuality, care and ageing; health and well-being of LGBT youth; and the needs and interests of older trans people.

1 Older Lesbian, Gay, Bisexual and Trans People

Minding the knowledge gaps

Andrew King, Kathryn Almack and Yiu-Tung Suen

Introduction

This book has two principal, but interconnected, aims: first, to address a series of knowledge gaps in the understanding of the lives of older lesbian, gay, bisexual and trans (LGBT) people; second, to bring a range of different authors together, emanating from academia, policy making, practice and activism, in order to address those gaps in knowledge.

The book arises from a project of the same name (referred to hereafter as the MTKG project), which was funded by the UK Economic and Social Research Council and ran from 2013 to 2015. The project, which was focused on knowledge gaps around LGBT ageing in the UK, was undertaken as a series of seven events: six seminars/workshops and a final, showcase conference. Each of the six seminars was composed of two presentations about an area of LGBT ageing where knowledge is lacking and then a workshop on how to address that area and the issues it raises. The final showcase conference, which took place in London, had presentations, panel discussions and workshop activities concerning the project, how to address knowledge gaps in the future, and the future of LGBT ageing research and practice in the UK. We discuss the project and its outcomes in more detail in the final chapter of this book. This book is therefore an artefact of that project, but it also represents a way of bringing together key writers in the field, considering new ways of approaching LGBT ageing and what practical applications could follow.

In this introductory chapter, we outline which knowledge gaps were focused on as part of the MTKG project, why they were chosen at the time and then discuss how the discrete chapters in this book will address them. We begin by setting the scene – explaining what knowledge gaps existed and why they were chosen as the basis for the project and this book. The chapter will then provide an overview of the structure of this book and how it is organised. Finally, we point to issues we return to in the final chapter of the book, which assess the value of the project we undertook, its limitations and what still needs to be done.

Finding the knowledge gaps

LGBT people aged 50 and over form a significant minority of the UK's ageing population (Department of Trade and Industry Women and Equality Unit, 2003; Price, 2005). Based on the commonly used estimate that 5 to 7 per cent of the UK population identifies as LGBT (Aspinall, 2009), Simpson et al. (Simpson et al., 2016) suggest that there are likely to be between 520,000 and 728,000 people, aged 65 and over, who are LGBT (using the UK 2011 Census figures for the total population aged 65 and over). While their experiences of ageing will have similarities with their cisgender and/or heterosexual peers, their lives will have been strongly and sometimes negatively affected by the social organisation of norms related to gender, gender identity and sexuality, what is commonly referred to in the academic literature as heteronormativity (Richardson, 2018). In this sense, as Almack (Chapter 11, p. 168, this volume) suggests, heteronormativity is:

> [A] cultural bias that views heterosexuality as 'normal' and taken for granted in a way that LGBT relationships and identities are not. Examples of heteronormativity include the under-representation of LGBT relationships and people in service promotion leaflets, or assumptions made that someone is heterosexual unless otherwise stated. Heteronormativity can make someone feel invisible, erase a big part of someone's identity, and impact on their ability to involve those closest to them in their care.

Indeed, writers suggest that heteronormativity will have particular significance for older LGBT adults who grew up in a more hostile, homophobic, biphobic and transphobic era than might currently be the case.[1] It may have left a lasting legacy of stigma and uncertainty, making people feel invisible and concerned about disclosing their identity to service providers and others, although it may also have created forms of resilience, such as group solidarity and self-efficacy (Blando, 2001; Rosenfeld, 2002; Persson, 2009; Fredriksen-Goldsen, 2011; Knauer, 2011; Witten, 2014; King, 2016).

Many studies, summarised previously in meta-analyses and anthologies (Fredriksen-Goldsen and Muraco, 2010; Witten and Eyler, 2012), have documented both the structural disadvantages faced by older LGBT adults, while also dispelling the myth of a lonely old age due to rejection by family and society. Studies have, for example, shown that older LGBT adults report higher rates of participation in non-familial social networks compared to their heterosexual counterparts (Brennan-Ing et al., 2013; Cronin and King, 2014). Nevertheless, concerns have been expressed about the absence of intergenerational support and reliance on single generational networks which grow smaller as one ages (Ward et al., 2012). Other studies, however, show how the provision of services, alongside the general experience of ageing, are often framed in accordance with stereotypical representations and understandings of sexuality and gender identity, which can adversely affect quality of life and health (for a good overview see Fish and Karban, 2015; Hudson-Sharp and Metcalf, 2016).

While there has been a growth in understanding around LGBT ageing over recent years, making knowledge gaps less obvious than before, when we commenced the MTKG project there were still areas, particularly in relation to how we understand LGBT ageing in the UK, that required more attention. Moreover, while we can draw upon a wide literature base to make postulations, especially using studies that emanate from other advanced industrial societies such as the USA, Canada and Australia, there are certain aspects of the UK context that make it both specific, as well as contributing to wider global debates. Thus, exploring knowledge gaps in LGBT ageing research in the UK remains important.

A range of legislative changes and policy initiatives took place in the UK during the early 2000s, which have challenged inequalities and discrimination as well as both encouraging and requiring organisations to engage with LGBT citizens (Mitchell et al., 2009; Richardson, 2018). The reorganization of local government, the personalisation agenda in health and welfare services and the advent of broader equality laws have arguably had a liberating effect on older LGBT people in ways that many never imagined would be possible. The introduction of, first, Civil Partnerships (2004) and, second, Same-Sex Marriage (2013) offered new ways of legally recognising relationships and benefits associated with such, including pension rights. Laws about the equal provision of goods and services, amalgamated in the Equality Act (2010), also meant that services related to housing, welfare and health should not discriminate against those from sexual and gender minority groups. The Gender Recognition Act (2004) enabled trans people to ensure that their birth certificate and other documents could reflect their authentic gender identity.[2] Again, all of these initiatives represented a considerable change in how the law and institutions treated LGBT people, certainly when compared to the pathologising and stigmatising of previous eras.

In many ways, research has developed considerably over the past decade to help our understanding about LGBT ageing and older people. Despite this, at the time the project started, little research existed in the UK on the lives of older bisexual men and women (Jones, 2011; Jones et al., 2018), or on the lives of older trans people (Bailey, 2012). Similarly, the experiences of older LGBT people from Black, Asian and minority ethnic (BAME) communities has been very much under-researched (Suen, 2015), in addition to older LGBT people who are less advantaged in terms of socio-economic status (Heaphy et al., 2004). It is important that research on LGBT ageing reflects diverse experiences and that the experiences of those who have been under-researched are fully taken into account. Indeed, a fundamental aim of the MTKG project was to include such voices, both as participants in the workshops/seminars and in the topics covered by them.

It is also clear that our knowledge of older LGBT people's experiences in certain policy debates and areas of practice has been either at a basic level or missing altogether. The significance of intergenerational diversity and dialogue, where different generations of LGBT people communicate and learn from one another, is an area that has had some limited research, but more could be undertaken (International Longevity Centre, 2011). Since 2008 and the coming of the global financial crisis, which affected the UK economy particularly significantly, there has been very little analysis of what effects this may have had on older LGBT people. Finally, areas within health and social care that require further study include: ageing with disabilities, end of life, dementia, and residential care (Almack, 2007; Almack et al., 2010; Westwood et al., 2015; Westwood, 2016).

Overall, despite knowledge gaps concerning older LGBT people narrowing over recent years, we contend that many remain and hence the reason why the MTKG project was necessary. Even now, in 2018, the topics covered by the project and in this book remain important and hence a collection such as this is timely.

Minding the gaps

Having identified a series of gaps in knowledge about LGBT ageing and older people, as well as a changing UK social, economic and political context, the MTKG project identified a number of key speakers who could address these gaps, create debate and, with an audience composed of academics, policy makers, practitioners, LGBT community members and activists, among others, look at ways in which gaps could be addressed and practical outcomes attained. In the final chapter of this book we report on each of those seminars/workshops, as well as the final, showcase conference. However, in the remainder of this chapter we want to draw attention to the structure of this book and the content of the chapters contained therein.

Chapters 2 and 3 both examine older bisexual lives. Rebecca L. Jones summarises what little is known about bisexuality and ageing. She identifies some potential solutions to address significant gaps in the evidence base about the lives of older bisexual people. These include: addressing how we theorise bisexuality; thinking more carefully about the significance of sexual identities in relation to sexual practices and sexual attractions; innovative research methodologies to capture the experiences and perspectives of older bisexual people; and different data analysis practices to ensure that the distinctiveness of bisexual experiences are not erased within LGBT research. Chapter 3 offers a reflexive account exploring why older people's bisexuality is so invisible and erased, as well as the effects of this on bisexual individuals. In this chapter, Sue George draws upon her own experiences and argues that the invisibility of older bi people can and must be challenged because – among other things – invisibility leads to the isolation of individuals, which in turn has a negative impact upon their mental health.

In Chapter 4, Louis Bailey, Jay McNeil and Sonja J. Ellis use data from the UK's largest survey of trans mental health to examine the mental health and well-being of older trans people, as well as their use of professional mental health services. Bailey et al. demonstrate that older trans people's mental health is complex – no single experience dominates, although they do suggest that, compared to trans individuals in other age groups, the older trans people they surveyed reported better rates of mental health compared to the general sample, in addition to higher rates of self-esteem and control over their lives. However, they caution against an overly optimistic viewpoint. Their data also demonstrates areas of concern, not least older trans people's experiences of formal mental health services, which shows areas for service improvement. Chapter 5, by Ruth Pearce, focuses attention on temporality and questions the linearity of ageing from a trans perspective. Drawing upon the notion of queer time (Halberstam, 2005), as well as her own research projects, Pearce illustrates how theories of trans temporality can help us understand the experiences and challenges faced by chronologically older trans people, while at the same time pointing to the need to queer temporality in relation to LGBT ageing.

Chapters 6 and 7 explore knowledge gaps around culture, ethnicity and religion. Chapter 6, by Joanne McCarthy and Roshan das Nair, employs intersectionality as a framework to view individuals as more than their sum of identities. It has been used successfully to develop a better understanding of people who inhabit multiple minority identities. They argue that the voices of older ethnic minority LGBT people are rarely heard, and review research that explores intersections of gender, sexuality, ethnicity and culture. They then take a specific focus on their own research that examined the experiences of older Irish gay men and the interaction between these identities and religion. In Chapter 7, Westwood, Suen and Scott identify and critically interrogate the absence of LGBT voices from the literature on BAME ageing and the absence of BAME voices from the literature on LGBT ageing. The chapter considers some of the reasons for those gaps, such as difficulty of accessing older BAME LGBT people, and the more fundamental question whether the LGBT identity labels are cross-culturally applicable for older people. It argues that there is a great need for research in this area, the agenda of which should be defined by older BAME LGBT people themselves, and that they should retain control of their stories and how they are heard.

Chapters 8 and 9 explore the issue of intergenerationality and LGBT ageing. Both chapters consider intergenerational projects that seek to bring older and younger LGBT people together. In Chapter 8, Dylan Kneale describes three innovative intergenerational LGB projects and the supporting evidence base that existed when they were developed. Kneale then considers new opportunities for quantitative research to enhance the evidence of need for intergenerational work among LGBT people in the UK, and presents the results from one such analysis. Kneale then explores how the evidence base for intergenerational work among LGBT people has developed since 2010/2011, before concluding that it is important that research on LGBT intergenerationality is accessible beyond academia, to policy makers and others. In Chapter 9, Catherine McNamara details a specific project, *IN-TERarts*, which involved working intergenerationally with people who identify as lesbian, gay, bisexual, trans and/or queer (LGBTQ). McNamara reflects on the specific challenges of working with a diversity of identities within intergenerational LGBTQ work. Indeed, *INTERarts* rejected a model of intergenerational work where older people provide stories and younger people create the artistic response, instead inviting stories from all participants and facilitating creative engagement with everyone. McNamara details how this challenged some established ideas in LGBTQ groups and also how new understandings about LGBTQ ageing were reached.

Chapters 10 and 11 move on to two under-researched and interrelated areas of LGBT ageing: residential care and end-of-life care. Chapter 10, by Paul Willis, Michele Raithby and Tracey Maegusuku-Hewett, critically explores some of the assumptions and meanings inherent in older lesbian and gay adults' discussions about preferred long-term care settings. While yet to be fully realised in the UK, specialist long-term care provision for older lesbian and gay adults is a growing phenomenon internationally; for example, 'LGBT'-specific retirement homes are operating in European nations, including France and Spain, and in some US states. Willis et al. present interview findings from a mixed-methods study into the provision of inclusive care environments for older lesbian and gay adults in Wales. They discuss how housing providers and social enterprises could explore and support the different models of housing provision identified by their research. In Chapter 11, Kathryn Almack provides a brief overview of end-of-life care in England and Wales, and goes on to address issues relating to end-of-life care for older LGBT people and the gaps in our knowledge in this area. Almack draws upon findings from the first major UK study of end-of-life care needs and experiences in the lives of older LGBT people, with a particular focus on concerns identified relating to care at home and care settings outside the home. Findings from this study suggest that diverse needs are not being met or are not offering adequate provision for older LGBT people. Health policy initiatives in England have encouraged providers at every stage of end-of-life care services to provide better coordinated and person-centred services, and Almack highlights the importance for services to be prepared to encounter LGBT people.

Since 2010, the British government has adopted a fiscal policy that has sought to reduce the budget deficit introducing a period of austerity. The two final substantive chapters in this collection consider the implications of this policy for older LGBT people and their experiences of ageing. In Chapter 12, Martin Mitchell, Mehul Kotecha and Malen Davies, from NatCen Social Research, outline the findings of two studies conducted in 2013 and 2016 for UNISON, the largest Trade Union in the UK covering the public sector. While not all LGBT older people were affected by public sector spending cuts, there were a number of ways in which they were, including making some feel isolated and marginalised. Moreover, evidence emerged that improving services for older LGBT was viewed, in some cases, as no longer affordable in times of austerity. This was without adequate alternative mainstream services and appropriate training for staff in those services being put in place. Similar evidence emerges in Chapter 13, in which Andrew King reflects on a project that sought to improve services used by older LGBT people. King outlines a project that sought to use LGBT ageing research and create an impact on those delivering services to older LGBT people. However, King notes that austerity shaped the project in a number of ways and he considers both the affective experiences of those involved and wider questions of LGBT citizenship that are invoked.

In Chapter 14, we focus attention on the MTKG project, the activities undertaken and the knowledge that was produced as a result. We also reflect on the gaps that the MTKG project failed to address or only did so partially and make recommendations for future work. Above all, we reflect back on the aims of the MTKG project and this collection. We argue that although the project advanced knowledge about LGBT ageing and older people, there is still important research, policy making and practice work still to do.

Notes

1 For instance, the partial decriminalisation of same-sex sexual acts between men occurred in 1967 in England and Wales; in Scotland in 1980, and in Northern Ireland in 1982. While female same-sex relationships were not criminalised, other sanctions held strong, such as removal of custody of children from lesbian parents which was still common in the 1970s

2 There have been a whole range of legislative changes in the UK since the early 2000s, which include the following: in 2001 the Age of Consent for gay men reduced to 16; in 2002 Equal Rights were granted to same-sex couples applying for adoption; 2003 saw the Repeal of Section 28 of the Local Government Act (1988) and the Employment Equality (Sexual Orientation) Regulations (2003) was passed, making it illegal to discriminate against lesbians, gay men and bisexuals in the workplace; in 2004 the Civil Partnership Act was passed, giving same-sex couples the same rights and responsibilities as married heterosexual couples; in 2004 the Gender Recognition Act enabled trans people to change their legal gender in the UK, allowing them to acquire a new birth certificate, affording them full recognition of their acquired sex in law for all purposes; in 2010 the Equality Act was passed, which includes the extension of the single public Equality Duty to cover LGBT people; in 2012 the Protection of Freedoms Act (2012) was passed, allowing for historic convictions for consensual gay sex to be removed from criminal records; in 2013 the Marriage (Same-Sex Couples) Act (2013) was passed in England and Wales; in 2014 the Scottish government passed legislation allowing same-sex couples to marry in Scotland.

References

Almack, K. (2007) 'Palliative Care and End of Life Care for the Non-heterosexual Community', *End of Life Care for Nurses*, 1(2): 27–32.
Almack, K., Seymour, J. and Bellamy, G. (2010) 'Exploring the Impact of Sexual Orientation on Experiences and Concerns about End of Life Care and on Bereavement for Lesbian, Gay and Bisexual Older People', *Sociology*, 44(5): 908–924.

Aspinall, PJ. (2009) *Estimating the size and composition of the lesbian, gay, and bisexual population in Britain.* Manchester: Equality and Human Rights Commission.

Bailey, L. (2012) 'Trans Ageing: Thoughts on a Life Course Approach in Order to Better Understand Trans Lives', in Ward, R., Rivers, I., and Sutherland, M. (eds) *Lesbian, Gay, Bisexual and Transgender Ageing: Biographical Approaches for Inclusive Care and Support,* London: Jessica Kingsley, pp. 51–66.

Blando, J. (2001) 'Twice Hidden: Older Gay and Lesbian Couples, Friends and Intimacy', *Generations,* 25(2): 87–89.

Brennan-Ing, M., Seidel, L., Larson, B. et al. (2013) 'Social Care Networks and Older LGBT Adults: Challenges for the Future', *Journal of Homosexuality,* 61(1): 21–52.

Cronin, A. and King, A. (2014) 'Only Connect? Lesbian, Gay and Bisexual (LGB) Adults and Social Capital', *Ageing and Society,* 34(2): 258–279.

Department of Trade and Industry Women and Equality Unit. (2003) *Civil Partnership: A Framework for the Legal Recognition of Same-sex Couples,* London: Department for Trade and Industry.

Fish, J. and Karban, K. (2015) *LGBT Health Inequalities: International Perspectives in Social Work,* Bristol: Policy Press.

Fredriksen-Goldsen, KI. (2011) 'Resilience and Disparities among Lesbian, Gay, Bisexual and Transgender Older Adults', *Public Policy and Aging Report,* 21(2): 3–7.

Fredriksen-Goldsen, KI. and Muraco, A. (2010) 'Aging and Sexual Orientation: A 25-year Review of the Literature', *Research on Aging,* 32(3): 372–413.

Halberstam, J. (2005) *In a Queer Time and Place: Transgender Bodies, Subcultural Lives,* New York: New York University Press.

Heaphy, B., Yip, AKT. and Thompson, D. (2004) 'Ageing in a Non-heterosexual Context', *Ageing and Society,* 24(6): 889–902.

Hudson-Sharp, N. and Metcalf, H. (2016) *Inequality among Lesbian, Gay Bisexual and Transgender Groups in the UK: A Review of Evidence,* London: National Institute for Economic and Social Research.

International Longevity Centre. (2011) *Celebrating Intergenerational Diversity Amongst LGBT People,* London: International Longevity Centre.

Jones, RL. (2011) 'Imagining Bisexual Futures: Positive, Non-normative Later Life', *Journal of Bisexuality,* 11(2–3): 245–270.

Jones, RL., Almack, K. and Scicluna, R. (2018) 'Older Bisexual People: Implications for Social Work from the "Looking Both Ways" Study', *Journal of Gerontological Social Work*: 1–14.

King, A. (2016) *Older Lesbian, Gay and Bisexual Adults: Identities, Intersections and Institutions,* London: Routledge.

Knauer, NJ. (2011) *Gay and Lesbian Elders: History, Law and Identity Politics in the United States,* Farnham: Ashgate.

Mitchell, M., Howarth, C., Kotecha, M. et al. (2009) *Sexual Orientation Research Review 2008,* Manchester: Equality and Human Rights Commission.

Persson, DI. (2009) 'Unique Challenges of Transgender Aging: Implications From the Literature', *Journal of Gerontological Social Work,* 52(6): 633–646.

Price, E. (2005) 'All but Invisible: Older Gay Men and Lesbians', *Nursing Older People,* 17(4): 16–18.

Richardson, D. (2018) *Sexuality and Citizenship,* Cambridge: Polity Press.

Rosenfeld, D. (2002) 'Identity Careers of Older Gay Men and Lesbians', in Gubrium, F. and Holstein, J. (eds), *Ways of Aging,* Oxford: Blackwell, pp. 160–181.

Simpson, P., Almack, K. and Walthery, P. (2016) '"We Treat Them All the Same": The Attitudes, Knowledge and Practices of Staff Concerning Old/er Lesbian, Gay, Bisexual and Trans Residents in Care Homes', *Ageing and Society* online-first. Available at www.cambridge.org/core/journals/ageing-and-society/article/ div-classtitlewe-treat-them-all-the-same-the-attitudes-knowledge-and-practices-of-staff-concerning-older-lesbian-gay-bisexual-and-trans-residents-in-care-hom esdiv/08C377AE4D1E23BB3E787E9BBC67F71E# (accessed 8 March 2018)(1–31).

Suen, Y-T. (2015) 'Lesbian, Gay, Bisexual and Transgender Ageing', in Twigg, J. and Martin, W. (eds), *Routledge Handbook of Cultural Gerontology,* London: Sage, pp. 226–233.

Ward, R., Rivers, I. and Sutherland, M. (2012) *Lesbian, Gay, Bisexual and Trans- gender Ageing: Biographical Approaches for Inclusive Care and Support*, London: Jessica Kingsley,

Westwood, S. (2016) 'Dementia, Women and Sexuality: How the Intersection of Ageing, Gender and Sexuality Magnify Dementia Concerns among Lesbian and Bisexual Women', *Dementia,* 15(6): 1494–1514.

Westwood, S., King, A., Almack, K. et al. (2015) 'Good Practice in Health and Social Care Provision for LGBT Older People', in Fish, J. and Karban, K. (eds), *Lesbian, Gay, Bisexual and Trans Health Inequalities,* Bristol: Policy Press, pp. 145–158.

Witten, TM. (2014) 'It's Not All Darkness: Robustness, Resilience, and Successful Transgender Aging', *LGBT Health,* 1(1): 24–33.

Witten, TM. and Eyler, AE. (2012) *Gay, Lesbian, Bisexual, and Transgender Aging: Challenges in Research, Practice, and Policy*, Baltimore, MD: Johns Hopkins Uni- versity Press.

2 Bisexual ageing

What do we know and why should we care?

Rebecca L. Jones

Introduction

Very little research focusing specifically on bisexual ageing has been conducted anywhere in the world. Ageing is a lifelong process so there is a small literature on the ageing experiences of bisexual people in their thirties, forties, fifties and early sixties, which this chapter overviews. However, there is an almost complete knowledge gap about bisexual people in their seventies, eighties or older. Studies of LGBTQ ageing more generally seldom offer meaningful information about the experiences of bisexual people as they grow older.

This chapter summarises what little is known about bisexuality and ageing, and identifies some of the most significant knowledge gaps. It then discusses four reasons for this lack of knowledge and some potential solutions which may help address these gaps. The reasons discussed are: understandings of bisexuality which work to minimise its prevalence and significance; oversimplifying the relationships between sexual identities, behaviours and attractions; data-collection and analysis practices which erase any distinctiveness to bisexual experiences; and difficulties finding research participants who are bisexual and older. The four corresponding potential solutions are: better theorisations of bisexuality; thinking more carefully about the significance of sexual identities in relation to sexual practices and sexual attractions; different data analysis practices; and alternative types of research. If the 'B' in LGBTQ is ever to be more than tokenistic, it is important that this knowledge gap is addressed. However, this chapter also argues that addressing the knowledge gaps around bisexuality and ageing can carry benefits for people of other sexualities in later life and for academics and practitioners interested in ageing or sexuality, by encouraging more sophisticated thinking about all sexual identities.

There are some commonalities between bisexual people and transgender, queer, intersex, asexual, etc. people in terms of their relative marginalisation within acronyms such as LGBT and LGBTQ (Barker et al., 2009). Bisexual people may also, of course, be transgender, queer, intersex or asexual and there is some evidence of significant overlap between bisexual and transgender and genderqueer communities (Barker et al., 2008, 2012).

There may also be some analogous reasons for knowledge gaps and similar potential solutions for these groups. However, these are beyond the scope of this chapter, which focuses specifically on bisexuality (for discussion of transgender ageing see Chapters 4 and 5, this volume, and for a rare focus on the intersection of bisexuality and transgender issues in later life see Witten, 2016). Bisexuality around the globe is also beyond the scope of this chapter, which focuses only on Anglophone Western cultures.

Defining bisexual ageing

Although this book is concerned with gaps in our knowledge about 'older' LGBT populations, it is also important to note that ageing is a lifelong process, not the property of people over a certain age (Bytheway, 2011; Twigg and Martin, 2015), and that experiences earlier in life continue to affect individuals as they grow older (Bengtson et al., 2005; Elder, 1974). Thus, 'bisexual ageing' in its broadest sense properly includes the ageing of bisexual people (a term defined below) at any stage of the life course. Bytheway (1995) argues that considering the ageing experiences of younger people can play an important role in reducing ageism and the 'othering' of older people. This project of reducing the 'othering' of older people is arguably especially important when older people are already stigmatised for other identity features, such as being black or minority ethnic, disabled and/or non-heterosexual.

However, there are some experiences which become much more common as people grow old, which mean that there is also merit in considering experiences of ageing in later life in particular. These common experiences in later life may include new expectations about social roles, encounters with ageism, retirement from any previous paid work and increased rates of certain disabilities and diseases such as arthritis.

This chapter therefore considers both the experiences of ageing of bisexual people of all ages and the experiences of bisexual people who are in some sense 'older' or 'old'.[1] Considering ageing as a lifelong process makes the arbitrariness of defining 'older' in relation to a particular chronological age especially apparent. However, it is worth noting that many studies of LGBTQ ageing start from the age of 50 or 55 (e.g. Guasp, 2011; Knocker, 2012; King, 2016).

'Bisexual' is often understood to reference sexual attraction to 'both men and women'. However, this chapter, in common with most work in the field of critical bisexuality (Monro, 2015), uses a definition which does not assume binary gender: 'attraction to more than one gender or attraction regardless of gender.' Some scholars of sexuality have recently suggested that the 'mostly straight' are a distinct group within the spectrum from heterosexuality to homosexuality (McCormack, 2018). For the purposes of this chapter, the 'mostly straight' (or 'Kinsey 1s') are within scope because the argument is about the inclusion of non-monosexual identities, rather than about the behaviours or experiences of particular groups of people. The term 'bisexual' is used here despite acknowledged difficulties and debates about the term (Ochs, 2007; Monro, 2015), and indeed with all sexual identity labels and categories (Foucault, 1976; Gosine, 2006), due to its greater familiarity than alternative terms such as 'pansexual' and 'middle sexualities'. Dictionary definitions of bisexuality (and homosexuality and heterosexuality) generally reference sexual attraction but sexual behaviour and sexual identity are more commonly used to recruit respondents to empirical studies, a distinction of particular salience to bisexual people, which will be discussed in more detail later in this chapter.

What do we know?

Knowledge takes multiple forms and is not limited to the outputs of empirical research studies. Much that is of use to practitioners and older bisexual people themselves can be discovered from the personal accounts of individual older bisexual people (as discussed in Chapter 3, this volume). There is also a small non-empirical literature written by practitioners and researchers with expertise in bisexuality, which suggests issues likely to affect older people. These include Keppel and Firestein's summaries of possible counselling issues for bisexual people in later life, such as 'coming out', isolation, lack of supportive networks, impacts of ageism, homophobia and biphobia (Keppel, 2006; Keppel and Firestein, 2007), and more general overviews of later life issues likely to affect older bisexual people (Dworkin, 2006; Rodriguez-Rust, 2012; Jones, 2016a). However, this chapter focuses more narrowly on knowledge gained from empirical research studies and published in peer-reviewed academic journals and books. Very little such empirical work has been carried out which focuses on the experiences of people with bisexual attractions, behaviours or identities as they grow older and barely any has yet been published which informs us significantly about the experiences of bisexual people over the age of 70.

Perhaps the most important study is Fredriksen-Goldsen et al.'s comparison of 174 bisexually identified cisgender survey respondents within their wider sample of 2,560 LGBT-identified people aged 50-plus living in the USA (Fredriksen-Goldsen et al., 2016). Their focus was on health equity and they found clear evidence that, controlling for other factors and compared to older lesbians and gay men, bisexual participants were in poorer mental and physical health. However, they found that this poorer health is attributable to four other factors: lower socio-economic status, higher internalised stigma, lower identity disclosure (being 'out') and less social support. This finding is important because it suggests that poorer health is not a result of being bisexual but of these mediating factors, which are amenable to change. They conclude:

> [O]ur findings support the idea that the accumulation of disadvantage results in persistent health inequities for bisexuals in older age.

The historical context of invisibility and rejection of bisexuality may limit access to resources across the life course, resulting by older age in more limited accumulation of wealth and health that supports optimal aging.

(Fredriksen-Goldsen et al., 2016, p. 475)

Weinberg et al.'s longitudinal study of a group of adults connected to the San Francisco Bisexual Centre focused more on questions of sexual identity and behaviour (Weinberg et al., 2001). The final wave of this study encountered the participants when they were aged 35 to 67 (average age 50), enabling the researchers to compare their experiences of bisexuality in mid-life to their experiences earlier in the life course. They found that most participants were having less sex with fewer partners. They were also more likely to be sexually active with only one gender – about one-fifth were having sex only with people of the same gender and about one-third only with people of a different gender. In addition, they were more likely to be monogamous later in life. Participants were also less connected to bisexual communities than they had previously been, in part due to the closure of the local Bisexual Centre. However, despite these changes, Weinberg et al. found that most participants' identities as bisexual were more stable in later life than they had been earlier in life. They argue that participants understood their sexual identity by looking back on their history of sexual relationships, rather than by focusing on current relationships.

More recently, Rowntree surveyed 67 Australian 'baby boomers' aged between 50 and 70 to explore the influences of ageing on their sexual expression (Rowntree, 2015). She asked respondents to mark their sexual orientation on a continuum from homosexual to heterosexual and 25 respondents reported themselves to be neither exclusively homosexual nor exclusively heterosexual. This study thus supplies useful information about older people who may not identify as bisexual but who do experience bisexual attractions and behaviours. Many of these respondents had previously been in conventional marriages but were experiencing later life very positively as a time when they could explore new possibilities and reappraise their own sexuality. Women were particularly open to the possibility of sexual relationships with other women in the future.

Schnarrs et al. (2016) undertook an online survey of bisexually identified people who identified as male, had had sex in the past year and whose last sexual partner was male – a relatively narrow definition of male bisexuality. Of their 2,833 respondents, approximately 27 per cent were aged over 50 and they compared their sexual experiences and behaviours to those of respondents aged under 50. They found that the older group were:

- less likely to use condoms;
- less likely to have anal sex;
- but more likely not to have used a condom if they did have anal sex;
- less likely to have had an HIV test in the past six months;

- more likely to report analingus;
- less likely to have had an orgasm (although the vast majority did);
- reported higher levels of pleasure and satisfaction.

They discuss ways in which these findings can be explained by what is already known about common changes to sexual behaviour and experience in later life; for example, that many older people report higher levels of sexual pleasure and satisfaction and that older people of all sexualities are less likely to have HIV tests than are younger people.

Witten (2016) focused on experiences and fears around ageing of people who identified as both bisexual and transgender. Fears around home care and being in residential care were especially prevalent. These fears centred on gender rather than on sexuality – they had little to say about bisexuality. Respondents had higher rates of disability and chronic illness than ageing trans lesbians.

In my own research I have employed creative methods (drawing and making collages) to enable bisexually identified adults (aged 20 to 66, mean 37.5) to imagine their own ageing and later life (Jones, 2011, 2012). Most participants imagined continuing bisexual identities and relatively positive visions of later life with many non-normative characteristics. In current work, undertaken with Kathryn Almack and Rachael Scicluna, we are analysing the findings of the *Looking Both Ways* study of 12 people aged 50-plus living in England with bisexual relationship histories.

The small size of the empirical literature on bisexual ageing in Anglophone Western nations, almost all of which is overviewed above, the diverse definitions of bisexuality and ageing employed, and the very different foci of these studies mean that it is challenging to draw conclusions about what is known. What does seem to be clear is that older bisexual people are at greater risk of being in poorer health (and also materially poorer) than lesbians and gay men, that connection to bisexual communities and other forms of social support can play a part in ageing well, and that bisexual people's sexual desires and behaviours continue to change and develop in later years.

What is not known?

Just as for lesbian and gay people, we do not have reliable baseline figures for the prevalence of bisexual attractions across the life course, let alone in later life. The sexologist Kinsey found very high rates of bisexual behaviour among adults (Kinsey et al., 1948, 1953) but did not have a representative sample of respondents. We do not know whether people become more or less likely to experience or express bisexual attractions as they grow older – there is some evidence of later life coming out as gay or lesbian once any adult children have left home or after the death or departure of a long-term partner (Fruhauf et al., 2009) – but we do not know whether this is also the case for people who identify as bisexual.

Bisexual older people are usually included in wider empirical studies of non-heterosexual ageing or LGBTQ ageing. However, the small proportion of bisexual respondents who are typically recruited, as well as the ways in which the data from these studies are collected, analysed and reported, means that little can be deduced about the specific experiences of bisexual older people, issues which will be discussed in more detail later in this chapter.

None of the empirical studies of bisexual ageing reported above had many respondents aged over 70 (and most had none). Thus we know little empirically about the experiences of bisexual people at the stage of life when they are more likely to encounter health difficulties and disabilities, and to draw more extensively upon health and social care services. There is a growing body of literature on how to make health and social care services more accessible to LGBTQ older people (Age Concern England, 2006; Rowan and Giunta, 2014; Westwood et al., 2015), some of which may be helpful to bisexual service users. However, there is little in these resources about the specific experiences and needs of bisexual people.

Little is known about the specific ageing experiences of older bisexual people with intersectional identity features such as being disabled, black or minority ethnic, or transgender. The small literature on the experiences of black and minority ethnic bisexual adults suggests that there are problems with racism and exclusion within bisexual and other LGBTQ communities (Yuen Thompson, 2012). It seems likely that such experiences of racism have particularly adverse effects on older non-white bisexual people, since racism becomes compounded with ageism.

Why do we know so little?

Many reasons might be suggested for why so little is known about bisexual ageing compared to lesbian and gay ageing. There has been a significant growth in many Anglophone and European countries over recent years in the political and cultural visibility of non-heterosexual sexualities, as well as increased levels of acceptance. However, this has been framed largely around lesbians and gay men, rather than around bisexuals (Richardson and Monro, 2012), as seen in the colloquial reduction of 'same-sex marriage' to 'gay marriage' (bisexual people may enter into same-sex marriages, but they do not become gay by doing so). It is therefore not surprising that research into ageing and later life replicates this wider tendency to focus on lesbians and gay men.

Underlying reasons for the lower visibility of bisexuality have been argued to include: the stigmatization of bisexual people as promiscuous and incapable of fidelity (Klein, 1993), the dismissal of bisexuality as a transitional or inauthentic sexuality (Barker and Langdridge, 2008), the systematic erasure of bisexuality (Richardson and Monro, 2012; San Francisco Human Rights Commission, 2010; Rodriguez-Rust, 2000b), 'monosexism' (the belief that attraction to one gender is better or more legitimate than attraction to more than one gender) (Nagle, 1995) and 'biphobia' (aversion towards bisexual people, a term introduced by Bennett (1992), and developed by Welzer-Lang (2008); see also Barker et al. (2012)). These culturally available resources for thinking about bisexuality naturally also influence researchers in ageing, who bear a responsibility to interrogate their own understandings and invocations of bisexuality.

In the following two sections, I focus more narrowly on four reasons for the knowledge gaps around bisexual ageing which seem particularly amenable to remedy by researchers. The four reasons are interlinked and are as follows:

1   Understandings of bisexuality that minimise its prevalence and significance.
2   Oversimplifying the relationships between sexual identities, sexual behaviours and sexual attractions.
3   Data categorisation and analysis practices that have the effect of erasing any distinctiveness to bisexual experience.
4   Difficulties recruiting research respondents who are both bisexual and older.

Understandings of bisexuality that minimise its prevalence and significance

How writers and researchers understand and theorise bisexuality (and also homosexuality and heterosexuality) is often not explicit in studies of LGBTQ ageing, especially in those which are not theoretically focused. This means that understandings of bisexuality can sometimes only be inferred from the ways in which categories are used and the consequences of research choices, rather than discussed directly. Some understandings of bisexuality, such as that it is always a transitional identity, have the effect of invalidating it as a legitimate sexual orientation altogether, as discussed above. Here, I discuss understandings of bisexuality which do allow for its validity but frame it in ways which have the effect of minimising bisexuality's significance and prevalence.

As Dobinson et al. note, 'much work that says it is about lesbian and bi women or gay and bi men is only about the same-sex sexual experiences or relationships of the bisexuals' (Dobinson et al., 2005, p. 44). Limiting the inclusion of bisexual people to their same-sex relationships tends to exclude monogamous bisexual people who are in different-sex relationships and, depending on the focus of the study, may also exclude single bisexual people (as well as some transgender and genderqueer people).

The implication of this practice seems to be that bisexual people are only included within categories such as 'LGB', 'LGBTQ' and 'non-heterosexual' in relation to their same-sex desires and practices. Their different-sex desires and practices seem to be understood as irrelevant or out-of-field. Theorists of bisexuality have argued that this positions bisexual people as 'half gay and half straight', to the detriment of their well-being and to the detriment of the viability of bisexuality as an identity (Weasel, 1996; Rodriguez-Rust, 2000b; Barker and Langdridge, 2008). Significantly, including bisexual people only in relation to their same-sex desires implies that bisexuality is being theorised as only ever a behaviour, never an identity.

Petford argues that bisexuality is often theorised as existing either in the past or in the future, but never in the present (Petford, 2003). In psychoanalytic literature, she argues, bisexuality is usually treated as something that should be left in the past in the journey towards monosexual maturity, whereas in Queer Theory bisexuality is often positioned as something that will feature in a utopian future when sexual identity labels will no longer be needed. This leaves little space for people to claim bisexual identities in the present.

Oversimplifying the relationships between sexual identities, behaviours and attractions

Scholars have long recognised that sexual identities do not map neatly on to sexual behaviours or sexual attractions for any sexuality (Plummer, 1995; Weeks, 2007) and vary by cultural, geographical and historical location (Foucault, 1976; Gosine, 2006). However, the relationship between sexual identities, behaviours and attractions is especially significant in relation to bisexuality, where they seem to be particularly poorly matched, with many more people reporting bisexual behaviours and attractions than identities (Jones, 2010, 2016b; Rodriguez-Rust, 2000a). This means that relying on self-identification as bisexual to recruit older people to research studies may lead to lower response rates than for older lesbians and gay men, thus contributing to knowledge gaps.

Research based in epidemiology, public health and sexual health often uses terminology based on behaviour rather than identity, thus talking about MSM (men who have sex with men) and, more rarely, WSW (women who have sex with women). However, this can obscure the distinctive experiences of bisexual people, unless the distinguishing terms MSMx (men who have sex with men exclusively) and MSMW (men who have sex with men and women) and WSWx and WSWM are used. Even the accurate use of labels which describe behaviour is sometimes undermined when identity labels are then imposed across behaviour categories. For example Sigma's long-running *Gay Men's Sex Surveys* do distinguish between MSMx and MSMW but the title suggests that the MSMW are somehow 'gay'. This may be due to underlying notions of bisexuality as 'half gay and half straight' as discussed above. The use of labels which describe behaviour rather than identity has also been argued to be problematic because of the ways in which this undervalues the significance of claimed identities and may obscure differences of sexual practice (Young and Meyer, 2005). Thus, focusing on sexual behaviours is also not adequate to capture the whole picture of bisexuality (or any sexuality) in later life.

Analytic practices

Studies of older LGBTQ people often analyse responses by the gender of participants rather than by their sexual identities. Thus, the experiences of bisexual men are considered alongside the experiences of gay men and those of bisexual women are considered alongside those of lesbians. This practice has been much critiqued by scholars of bisexuality (Barker et al., 2012; Monro, 2015; Brotman et al., 2002; Welzer-Lang, 2008), who argue that it obscures differences between lesbians and bisexual women and gay and bisexual men, and contributes to the silencing of bisexuality as a legitimate sexual identity. It implies that bisexual people are understood to be 'half gay and half straight', since their 'gay' experiences may be elided with those of lesbians and gay men. It also means that even though bisexual people took part in a study, nothing can be discovered about what is distinctive to bisexual experience. Given that bisexual respondents are usually a small minority, this practice makes it impossible to claim with any certainty that the findings also hold true for bisexual (or transgender or queer) older people.

Difficulties recruiting respondents

Researchers often use identity labels to recruit respondents to studies of LGBTQ ageing, since they may provide a shorthand summary of initial inclusion criteria and may also encourage participation and a sense of shared ownership, especially when researchers also identify with that label (Jones, 2016b). As already discussed, the identity label 'bisexual' reaches only a small proportion of those people who experience attractions to more than one gender. It is not clear whether the label 'bisexual' is particularly problematic in recruiting older people rather than younger or midlife people – the prominence of bisexuality has varied over the lifetimes of currently 'older' people but it is worth noting that it came into more everyday use in the 1920s and was highly visible in the 1970s (Ochs and Highleyman, 2000), so it is not a new term.

In addition, the relatively small size of bisexual communities and scarcity of bi-inclusive spaces and venues, compared to larger lesbian and, especially, gay communities and spaces (Monro, 2015), makes it much more challenging to recruit bisexual people to any study. When researching older lesbian, gay, bisexual or transgender people, the ageism found in many venues and communities creates additional barriers (Ward et al., 2008) but these are especially stark given the small size of bisexual communities to start with. For example, while there are now many well-established groups for older LGBTQ people in the UK, they are largely made up of lesbian- and gay-identified participants (although many will have had relationships with more than one gender over the course of their lives). Opportunities for older bisexuals in the UK to meet together in a group to talk about ageing are currently limited to occasional workshops at community events and one monthly London group with a small membership.

How could we change this?

Wider societal change reducing biphobia and legitimising bisexuality as an authentic sexuality would doubtless contribute to reducing knowledge gaps around bisexual ageing. However, this section, as with the previous one, focuses on changes that could be made by individual researchers and groups of researchers, rather than those that require much wider societal and political change. Mirroring the four reasons identified above, four potential solutions are discussed here that would help reduce the knowledge gaps around bisexuality in later life. They are as follows:

1   Better theorisations of bisexuality.
2   Thinking more carefully about the relationships of sexual identities, behaviours and attractions.
3   Different data analysis practices.
4   Alternative types of research.

Better theorisations of bisexuality

Better theorisations of bisexuality have the potential to reduce knowledge gaps by offering ways of interrogating bisexuality in later life that take bisexuality seriously as a sexual identity, behaviour and attraction, and include more bisexual people (not just those in same-sex relationships).

Perhaps the most comprehensive recent overview of bisexuality is found in Surya Monro's monograph *Bisexuality: Identities, Politics, and Theories* (2015). This book is particularly useful in its attempt to make connections between the relatively small literature focusing particularly on bisexuality and the much wider literature on sexuality and feminism, queer theory, sociology and political science. An older but more encyclopaedic collection is Paula Rodriguez-Rust's *Bisexuality in the United States: A Social Science Reader* (Rodriguez-Rust, 2000a) which contains chapters on a wide range of different aspects of bisexuality. Beth Firestein's collection *Becoming Visible: Counseling Bisexuals across the Lifecourse* (Firestein, 2007) offers a useful practitioner-focused summary likely to be of interest to people working in a variety of fields beyond counselling and therapies.

There is also a body of more theoretical work on bisexuality, often drawing upon or responding to queer theory, and attempting to think carefully about the differences between bisexual identities and other sexual identities

(James, 1996; Bi Academic Intervention, 1997; Storr, 1999; Hemmings, 2002; Gurevich et al., 2007; Klesse, 2007). There is some evidence that certain people's bisexual identities are more fluid and changeable than many people's lesbian and gay identities (Rodriguez-Rust, 2007; Diamond, 2008). However, the evidence for this is strongest in relation to women, and specifically young women – it is not so strong for men and for older people. These theorisations of bisexuality can be drawn upon by scholars of LGBTQ ageing to enable the better inclusion of bisexual people within studies of wider LGBTQ ageing.

Thinking more carefully about the relationships of sexual identities, behaviours and attractions

Researchers planning and undertaking studies of LGBTQ ageing could ask themselves whether identities, behaviours or attractions were relevant to the research questions of a particular study, and then either try to avoid or at least note slippage between the three. Researchers might also rethink recruitment practices so that they depended less on people identifying as bisexual, which may then able them to recruit a wider range of types of bisexual people as well as a greater number. Rowntree's study of baby boomers discussed above (Rowntree, 2015) suggests one such approach – recruiting from the whole population and then using a continuum to identify sexual orientation. The *Looking Both Ways* study I am currently leading set out specifically to recruit older people with a history of relationships with more than one gender but who did not currently identify as bisexual, as well as those who did (Jones et al., 2016). Such an approach, of course, needs to be careful not to claim that participants are in some sense 'really' bisexual. However, it may shed useful light both on why people with similar relationship histories choose different sexual identity labels and on issues arising in later life for people with these kinds of relationship histories.

Different data analysis practices

Barker et al. have produced a set of good practice guidelines for researchers and writers on bisexuality (Barker et al., 2012). The first of these is 'Separate bisexuals from the other groups' (p. 385). Almack's study of end-of-life care and older LGBT people (see Chapter 11, this volume) provides an example of this approach, which provides information about bisexuality in later life, as does the paper by Fredriksen-Goldsen et al. discussed above. Secondary analysis of existing datasets can also play a useful role here. Colledge et al. reanalysed a dataset which had previously amalgamated the responses of lesbians with those of bisexual women, and found statistically significant differences between the two groups (Colledge et al., 2015). This provided valuable information about the distinctive health needs and experiences of bisexual women. It also disproved the notion that the responses of bisexual people cannot be considered separately because numbers are too small. This approach could also be taken with existing datasets focusing on LGBTQ ageing and later life. Where numbers of bisexual respondents are very small, amalgamating the responses of bisexual men with those of bisexual women may make it possible to characterise distinctive features of bisexual experiences of ageing. Genderqueer bisexual participants could also be properly included in a study taking this approach, rather than being either left out or miscategorised. Doing so would also have the benefit of privileging sexual identity over gender as the lens through which sexuality is read (Gurevich et al., 2007).

Alternative types of research

While there is no easy way to 'find' significant numbers of bisexual older people, genuinely participative and community-based types of research (Hagger-Johnson et al., 2006) may offer some help. If older bisexual people are involved in the design, implementation and/or analysis of research, this may help increase response rates to a study, as well as carrying important benefits to the project itself. Hagger-Johnson et al. (2013) argue for the particular importance of participative and community-based types of research when working with sexual communities that have been stigmatised. They argue that participative and community-driven research are essential if the knowledge of academics is to be joined to the expertise of others, in ways that are both academically rigorous and useful and/or emancipatory. This argument seems especially applicable to research into the experiences of older bisexual people, and is likely to be essential for older bisexual people encountering additional issues such are racism, ill-health or disability, or transphobia.

An alternative solution to the 'problem' of recruiting sufficient numbers of older bisexual people is to undertake different types of research which do not rely so much on number of participants to ensure validity and rigor; for example, case study research (Yin, 2003), narrative analysis (Riessman, 1993), discourse analysis (Edwards and Potter, 1992), conversation analysis (Sacks, 1995) and other such approaches.

Why should we care?

Researchers and practitioners working with lesbian and gay older people have built up a significant body of knowledge and good practice, albeit still limited and with its own knowledge gaps. This body of knowledge may be drawn upon both by specialist practitioners and those providing generic older people's services, in order to improve the lives of older lesbians and gay men. The absence of such a body of knowledge in relation to bisexual (and transgender, queer and so on) older people means that they are less likely to encounter services and support which are sensitive to their particular life experiences, especially if these experiences and needs differ from those of lesbians and gay men. Brotman et al. (2002) found that bisexual participants were more likely than lesbian or gay participants to experience difficulties with health care providers because of those providers' lack of understanding of their sexuality. Increased rates of health care encounters in later life mean that difficulties accessing appropriate and sensitive health care may be a particular issue for bisexual people as they grow older.

More theoretically, studying ageing and bisexuality brings into sharp focus the distinctions between sexual identity, sexual attraction and sexual behaviour, and the fact that they may not map neatly on to one another. This also draws our attention to the fact that not everyone who experiences exclusively same-sex attractions identifies as gay or lesbian, since these terms are often more available to white, Anglophone and middle-class people (Gosine, 2006). It reminds us that the group of older people who are usually reached by studies of LGBTQ ageing – those who do identify as L, G, B, T or Q to some extent, and are connected to LGBTQ organisations – may be very different from other exclusively same-sex-attracted older people. Thus we should care about bisexuality and ageing because it helps us to also think more carefully and inclusively about the ageing of those who are only same-sex attracted as well. The distinctions between sexual identity, attraction and behaviour may also be usefully applied to heterosexual older people, and to sexual practices, rather than just sexual orientations. These distinctions also have practical implications, for example, in the terminology used to devise sexual and general health information and to advertise activities and groups for older people.

Addressing some of the knowledge gaps around bisexual ageing could also carry benefits to people interested in ageing and later life. Studies of people with bisexual histories can make particularly clear the effects of significant life course events on later life, making more appropriate and personalised care possible (Jones, 2016b). Studies of bisexual older people can also make clear the heterogeneity of older people, and the ways in which ageing is being reshaped in the twenty-first century (Twigg and Martin, 2015). Studies of older bisexual people may also illuminate further the historical and cultural contingency of the claiming of any sexual or gender identity (Foucault, 1976; Gosine, 2006).

Perhaps most fundamentally, we should care about the lack of knowledge about bisexual ageing in terms of simple equity within the umbrella terms 'LGBT', 'LGBTQ' and so on. If 'B' is part of the acronym, then bisexuality should surely also be a fully considered part of a research project (as also should 'T' and 'Q' and any further letters employed). Better, perhaps, to specify that research is only into the experiences of lesbians and gay men than to claim LGBT or LGBTQ for research which is really only focused on lesbians and gay men. But better still to undertake research which treats bisexuality as a legitimate and autonomous sexual identity, thereby contributing to a more nuanced and sophisticated understanding of all sexualities in later life.

Note

1 However, studies of younger bisexual people which differentiate between age groups but do not focus on issues of ageing and later life are not within the scope of this chapter.

References

Age Concern England (2006) *The Whole of Me: Meeting the Needs of Older Lesbians, Gay Men and Bisexuals Living in Care Homes and Extra Care Housing. A Resource Pack for Professionals*. London: Age Concern England.

Barker, M. and Langdridge, D. (2008) 'Bisexuality: Working with a silenced sexuality', *Feminism & Psychology*, 18(3): 389–394.

Barker, M., Richards, C. and Bowes-Catton, H. (2009) '"All the world is queer save thee and ME [...]": Defining queer and bi at a Critical Sexology Seminar', *Journal of Bisexuality*, 9(3–4): 363–379.

Barker, M., Bowes-Catton, H., Iantaffi, A., Cassidy, A. and Brewer, L. (2008) 'British bisexuality: A snapshot of bisexual identities in the UK', *Journal of Bisexuality*, 8(1–2): 141–162.

Barker, M., Yockney, J., Richards, C., Jones, RL., Bowes-Catton, H. and Plowman, T. (2012) 'Guidelines for researching and writing about bisexuality', *Journal of Bisexuality*, 12(3): 376–392.

Bengtson, VL., Elder, GHJ. and Putney, NM. (2005) 'The lifecourse perspective on ageing: Linked lives, timing and history', in Johnson, ML. (ed.), *The Cambridge Handbook of Age and Ageing*. Cambridge: Cambridge University Press, pp. 9–17.

Bennett, K. (1992) 'Feminist bisexuality: A both/and option for an either/or world', in Weise, ER. (ed.), *Close to Home: Bisexuality and Feminism*. Seattle, WA: Seal Press, pp. 205–231.

Bi Academic Intervention (1997) The Bisexual Imaginary: Representation, Identity and Desire. London: Cassell.

Brotman, S., Ryan, BW., Jalbert, Y. and Rowe, B. (2002) 'The impact of coming out on health and health care access', *Journal of Health & Social Policy*, 15(1): 1–29.

Bytheway, B. (1995) *Ageism*. Buckingham: Open University Press.

Bytheway, B. (2011) Unmasking Age: The Significance of Age for Social Research. Bristol: Policy Press.

Colledge, L., Hickson, F., Reid, D. and Weatherburn, P. (2015) 'Poorer mental health in UK bisexual women than lesbians: Evidence from the UK 2007 Stonewall women's health survey', *Journal of Public Health*, 37(3): 1–11.

Diamond, LM. (2008) *Sexual Fluidity: Understanding Women's Love and Desire*. Cambridge, MA: Harvard University Press.

Dobinson, C., Macdonnell, J., Hampson, E., Clipsham, J. and Chow, K. (2005) 'Improving the access and quality of public health services for bisexuals', *Journal of Bisexuality*, 5(1): 41–78.

Dworkin, SH. (2006) 'Aging bisexual: The invisible of the invisible minority', in Kimmel, D., Rose, T. and David, S. (eds), *Lesbian, Gay, Bisexual and Transgender Aging: Research and Clinical Perspectives*. New York: Columbia University Press.

Edwards, D. and Potter, J. (1992) *Discursive Psychology*. London: Sage.

Elder, GH. (1974) Children of the Great Depression: Social Change in Life Experiences. Chicago, IL: University of Chicago Press.

Firestein, B. (2007) *Becoming Visible: Counselling Bisexuals across the Lifespan.* New York: Columbia University Press.

Foucault, M. (1976) The History of Sexuality: Volume 1: An Introduction. London: Allen Lane.

Fredriksen-Goldsen, KI., Shiu, C., Bryan, AEB., Goldsen, J. and Kim, H-J. (2016). 'Health equity and aging of bisexual older adults: Pathways of risk and resilience', *The Journals of Gerontology: Series B*, 72(3):468–478.

Fruhauf, CA., Orel, NA. and Jenkins, DA. (2009) 'The coming-out process of gay grandfathers: Perceptions of their adult children's influence', *Journal of GLBT Family Studies*, 5(1–2): 99–118.

Gosine, A. (2006) '"Race", culture, power, sex, desire, love: Writing in "men who have sex with men"', *IDS Bulletin*, 37(5): 27–33.

Guasp, A. (2011) Lesbian, Gay and Bisexual People in Later Life. London: Stonewall.

Gurevich, M., Bower, J., Mathieson, CM. and Dhayanandhan, B. (2007) '"What do they look like and are they among us?": Bisexuality, (dis)closure and (un)viability', in Clarke, V. and Peel, E. (eds), *Out in Psychology: Lesbian, Gay, Bisexual, Trans and Queer Perspectives*. London: Wiley-Blackwell, pp. 217–241.

Hagger-Johnson, G., Hegarty, P., Barker, M. and Richards, C. (2013) 'Public engagement, knowledge transfer and impact validity', *Journal of Social Issues*, 69(4): 664–683.

Hagger-Johnson, GE., McManus, J., Hutchinson, C., and Barker, M. (2006) 'Building partnerships with the voluntary sector', *The Psychologist*, 19(3): 156–158.

Hemmings, C. (2002) *Bisexual Spaces: A Geography of Sexuality and Gender.* New York and London: Routledge.

James, C. (1996) 'Denying complexity: The dismissal and appropriation of bisexuality in Queer, lesbian and gay theory', in Beemyn, B. and Eliason, M. (eds), *Queer Studies: Lesbian, Gay, Bisexual and Transgender Anthology*. New York: New York University Press, pp. 217–240.

Jones, RL. (2010) 'Troubles with bisexuality in health and social care', in Jones, RL. and Ward, R. (eds.), *LGBT Issues: Looking beyond Categories*. Edinburgh: Dunedin Academic Press, pp. 42–55.

Jones, RL. (2011) 'Imagining bisexual futures: Positive, non-normative later life', *Journal of Bisexuality*, 11(2–3): 245–270.

Jones, RL. (2012) 'Imagining the unimaginable: Bisexual roadmaps for ageing', in Ward, R., Rivers, I. and Sutherland, M. (eds), *Lesbian, Gay, Bisexual and Transgender Ageing: Biographical Approaches for Inclusive Care and Support*. London: Jessica Kingsley, pp. 21–38.

Jones, RL. (2016a) 'Aging and bisexuality', in Goldberg, A. (ed.), *The SAGE Encyclopaedia of LGBTQ Studies*. London: Sage.

Jones, RL. (2016b) 'Sexual identity labels and their implications in later life: The case of bisexuality', in Peel, E. and Harding, R. (eds), *Ageing & Sexualities: Interdisciplinary Perspectives*. Farnham: Ashgate, pp. 97–118.

Jones, RL., Almack, K. and Scicluna, R. (2016) *Ageing and Bisexuality: Case Studies from the 'Looking Both Ways' Project*. Milton Keynes: The Open University.

Keppel, B. (2006) 'Affirmative psychotherapy with older bisexual women and men', *Journal of Bisexuality*, 6(1–2): 85–104.

Keppel, B. and Firestein, B. (2007) 'Bisexual inclusion in addressing issues of GLBT aging: Therapy with older bisexual women and men', in Firestein, B. (ed.),

Becoming Visible: Counselling Bisexuals across the Lifespan. New York: Columbia University Press, pp. 164–185.

King, A. (2016) *Older Lesbian, Gay and Bisexual Adults: Identities, Intersections and Institutions*. London: Routledge.

Kinsey, AC., Pomeroy, WB. and Martin, CE. (1948) *Sexual Behavior in the Human Male*. London: WB. Saunders and Co.

Kinsey, AC., Pomeroy, WB., Martin, CE. and Gebhard, PH. (1953) *Sexual Behavior in the Human Female*. London: WB. Saunders and Co.

Klein, F. (1993) *The Bisexual Option*. New York: Haworth Press.

Klesse, C. (2007) *The Spectre of Promiscuity: Gay Male and Bisexual Non-monogamies and Polyamories*. Aldershot: Ashgate.

Knocker, S. (2012) *Perspectives on Ageing: Lesbians, Gay Men and Bisexuals*. York: Joseph Rowntree Foundation.

McCormack, M. (2018) 'Mostly straights and the study of sexualities: An introduction to the special issue', *Sexualities*, 21(1–2): 3–15.

Monro, S. (2015) *Bisexuality: Identities, Politics and Theories*. London: Palgrave Macmillan.

Nagle, J. (1995) 'Framing radical bisexuality: Toward a gender agenda', in Tucker, N. (ed.), *Bisexual Politics: Theories, Queries, and Visions*. Binghamton, NY: Harrington Park Press.

Ochs, R. (2007) 'What's in a name? Why women embrace or resist bisexual identity', in Firestein, BA. (ed.), *Becoming Visible: Counseling Bisexuals across the Lifespan*. New York: Columbia University Press, pp. 72–86.

Ochs, R. and Highleyman, L. (2000) 'Bisexual movement', in Zimmerman, B. (ed.), *Lesbian Histories and Cultures: An Encyclopedia*. London: Routledge, pp. 112–114.

Petford, B. (2003) 'Power in the darkness: Some thoughts on the marginalisation of bisexuality in psychological literature', *Lesbian and Gay Psychology Review*, 4(2): 5–13.

Plummer, K. (1995) Telling Sexual Stories: Power, Change and Social Worlds. London: Routledge.

Richardson, D. and Monro, S. (2012) *Sexuality, Equality and Diversity*. Basingstoke: Palgrave Macmillan.

Riessman, CK. (1993) *Narrative Analysis*. London: Sage.

Rodriguez-Rust, PC. (2000a) *Bisexuality in the United States: A Social Science Reader*. New York: Columbia University Press.

Rodriguez-Rust, PC. (2000b) 'Preface', in Rodriguez-Rust, PC. (ed.), *Bisexuality in the United States: A Social Science Reader*. New York: Columbia University Press.

Rodriguez-Rust, PC. (2007) 'The construction and reconstruction of bisexuality: Inventing and reinventing the self', in Firestein, BA. (ed.), *Becoming Visible: Counseling Bisexuals across the Lifespan*. New York: Columbia University Press, pp. 3–27.

Rodriguez-Rust, PC. (2012) 'Aging in the bisexual community', in Witten, TM. and Eyler, AE. (eds), *Gay, Lesbian, Bisexual and Transgender Aging: Challenges in Research, Practice and Policy*. Baltimore, MD: The Johns Hopkins University Press, pp. 162–186.

Rowan, NL. and Giunta, N. (2014) 'Special Issue: Lesbian, gay, bisexual, and transgender (LGBT) aging: The role of gerontological social work', *Journal of Gerontological Social Work*, 57(2–4): 75–406.

Rowntree, MR. (2015) 'The influence of ageing on baby boomers' not so straight sexualities', *Sexualities*, 18(8): 980–996.

Sacks, H. (1995) *Lectures on Conversation*. Oxford: Blackwell.

San Francisco Human Rights Commission (2010) *Bisexual Invisibility: Impacts and Recommendations*. San Francisco, CA: San Francisco Human Rights Commission LGBT Advisory Committee.

Schnarrs, PW., Rosenberger, JG. and Novak DS. (2016) 'Differences in sexual health, sexual behaviors, and evaluation of the last sexual event between older and younger bisexual men', *Journal of Bisexuality*, 16(1): 41–57.

Storr, M. (1999) *Bisexuality: A Critical Reader*. London: Routledge.

Twigg, J. and Martin, W. (2015) 'The challenge of cultural gerontology', *The Gerontologist*, 55(3): 353–359.

Ward, R., Jones, R., Hughes, J., Humberstone, N. and Pearson, R. (2008) 'Intersections of ageing and sexuality: Accounts from older people', in Ward, R. and Bytheway, B. (eds), *Researching Age and Multiple Discrimination*. London: Centre for Policy on Ageing, pp. 45–72.

Weasel, LH. (1996) 'Seeing between the lines: Bisexual women and therapy', *Women & Therapy*, 19(2): 5–16.

Weeks, J. (2007) The World We Have Won: The Remaking of Erotic and Intimate Life. London: Routledge.

Weinberg, MS., Williams, CJ. and Pryor, DW. (2001) 'Bisexuals at midlife: Commitment, salience and identity', *Journal of Contemporary Ethnography*, 30(2): 180–208.

Welzer-Lang, D. (2008) 'Speaking out loud about bisexuality: Biphobia in the gay and lesbian community', *Journal of Bisexuality*, 8(1–2): 81–95.

Westwood, S., King, A., Almack, K., Suen, Y-T. and Bailey, L. (2015) 'Good practice in health and social care provision for older LGBT people', in Fish, J. and Karban, K. (eds), *Social Work and Lesbian, Gay, Bisexual and Trans Health Inequalities: International Perspectives*. Bristol: Policy Press, pp. 145–158.

Witten, TM. (2016) 'Aging and transgender bisexuals: Exploring the intersection of age, bisexual sexual identity, and transgender identity', *Journal of Bisexuality*, 16(1): 58–80.

Yin, RK. (2003) *Case Study Research: Design and Methods*. Thousand Oaks, CA: Sage.

Young, RM. and Meyer, IH. (2005) 'The trouble with "MSM" and "WSW": Erasure of the sexual-minority person in public health discourse', *American Journal of Public Health*, 95(7): 1144–1149.

Yuen Thompson, B. (2012) 'The price of "community" from bisexual/biracial women's perspectives', *Journal of Bisexuality*, 12(3): 417–428.

3 You're not *still* bisexual, are you?

Bi identity, community and invisibility, moving towards and in older age

Sue George

Introduction

There has been very little written on the needs, interests and issues concerning people over 50 years of age who identify as bisexual, relate to that label in some way, or have bisexual relationship histories. Why are older bisexuals invisible in, or actively erased from, discussions on sexuality, or about older people? What, indeed, are our needs and concerns? Who, even, are we – us bisexual people over 50? Given that I am well into that age range and have identified as bisexual since 1973, these are matters of increasing urgency for me.

In this chapter, more reflexive and informal than many in this book, I will consider some of these issues. These observations and reflections will be filtered through the prism of my own experience and writings, and will include findings from my own small-scale, informal or journalistic research over that time. But while this chapter is personal rather than academic, it refers to theory where relevant. It also comes from a British perspective which is subtly different from the much more developed US bi movement, and focuses on UK-based experiences. Rather than research-based – although it refers to research in those very few areas where it exists – it incorporates discussions and interviews with others for whom the identity 'bisexual' is significant, whether or not it is one they wholly accept for themselves.

Bi visibility – for younger people

Young bisexual people – those under 40 – are now more visible in popular culture and the media than ever before. From celebrities announcing their sexuality, to Twitter hashtags, or Huffington Post features on "the most annoying questions people ask bisexuals", bisexuality is far more visible than it was ten or more years ago.

At the same time, various surveys show that increasing numbers of younger people 'don't identify as 100 per cent heterosexual'. Research carried out in the UK by YouGov, and using the Kinsey Scale, shows that 43 per cent of respondents aged 18 to 24 identified as neither wholly heterosexual nor homosexual, while corresponding percentages for those aged 25 to 39, 40 to 59 and 60-plus were 29 per cent, 16 per cent and 7 per cent respectively (YouGov, 2015). A similar survey indicated that one-third of Americans under 30 identified as other than 100 per cent heterosexual, with 16 per cent saying they are bisexual in some way (YouGov US, 2015). This seems like a big change.

So what about older bisexuals? Where are the 7 per cent of older British people who identified as bi in these surveys, or others for whom the label *bisexual* remains relevant in some way? Bi people over age 50 remain largely invisible and there seems to be a widespread assumption that only younger people identify as bisexual.

This assumption is tied in with the stereotypical beliefs that bisexuality is only connected with sexual and emotional experimentation, having fun, to the period before 'settling down'. For many, the 'sex' in 'bisexual' appears to be of prime importance. However, the bi community generally accepts the definition on the website of long-time US bisexual activist Robyn Ochs.

> I call myself bisexual because I acknowledge that I have in myself the potential to be attracted – romantically and/or sexually – to people of more than one sex and/or gender, not necessarily at the same time, not necessarily in the same way, and not necessarily to the same degree.
>
> (http://robynochs.com/bisexual/)

While also agreeing with Ochs' definition, my feelings about my own bisexuality go further than that. For me, identifying as bisexual goes far beyond my own sexual or romantic behaviour now, or in the past few years. For me, bisexuality encompasses desire, fantasy, relationship to mainstream society, politics, history, assumptions about people, close friendships and friendship networks, and my place in the world. For me, my bisexuality is about my whole self, and my whole life. This view of bisexuality has endured no matter what my relationships at any given point in time, including one partnership that lasted several decades.

A brief history of (bi) sexuality

So if it is the case that many fewer people born before – as a random cut-off point – 1966 currently identify as bi, why is this the case? The answer to this is complex and unclear. Bisexuality is not a new identity, but the barriers to recognising those feelings in oneself, or acting on them, used to be much higher and this may have an impact upon how older people see themselves now.

During the early part of the twentieth century, same-sex relationships (whether between men or women) were considered always wrong and, for men, illegal. Sex between men was partially decriminalised in 1967 (in England and Wales; later in the other UK nations). Nevertheless, some people had same-sex relationships (Porter and Weeks, 1990; Houlbrook, 2005) and a few of them did explicitly define as bisexual (Shute, 1931; Wolff, 1977; Shute, 1992), although how far this was the case outside of bohemian circles is hard to tell. At the same time, sexual relationships between men and women were considered 'natural' albeit highly policed (Szreter and Fisher, 2010). This began to liberalise to some extent in the 1960s, when contraception became more readily available and sex outside marriage was more accepted.

The theories of sexual liberation that came out of the late 1960s led to the women's liberation movement, and gay liberation, all of which were significant for bisexuality. The women's liberation movement wanted to challenge everything about the way women's lives were constructed at that time, including the supremacy of the nuclear family, the way children were brought up, and the way men and women related to each other. These feminists forefronted their friendships with other women, and this closeness sometimes led to same-sex relationships. Gay liberation wanted to get rid of categories of sexuality and gender, and challenged society's norms through dramatic interventions and communal living. Initially, some of these 'gay libbers' had sex with men and women, but this became considered a lack of commitment to the cause (Power, 1995).

Bisexuality first gained publicity at this time, thanks to David Bowie's proclamations that he was bisexual himself. This was the first of many times bisexuality was called 'trendy'. My own memory of the mid- to late 1970s was that bisexuality was relatively acceptable in the leftist feminist circles in which I moved; the first serious book on the subject was published in the UK in 1977 (Wolff).

However, in the early 1980s, the lesbian separatist current became more influential within feminism. Women were divided into two distinct categories – lesbian and heterosexual – and lesbianism, as a political choice, was considered the superior one. Bi women were often unwelcome in the lesbian community – after all, surely we would 'go off with men' – and many of us felt guilty that we could not be lesbians. When bi women were acknowledged at all, our sexuality was considered inherently problematic. Some bi women were part of the lesbian community and ignored or repressed their non-lesbian feelings (George, 1993, esp. pp. 38–64). In the early 1990s, this separatism began to lose influence and some women actively rejected it in favour of a more 'sex-positive' lesbianism. Nevertheless, its influence remains for many older women, whether or not they do or have ever identified as lesbian.

The situation for men was different. A commercial gay scene developed in many areas during the 1970s, but the HIV/AIDS epidemic of the early 1980s onward had a terrible impact upon gay and bi men – both upon their own health and lives, and upon the increase in homophobia. The introduction into law of Section 28 in 1988 – which prohibited the "promotion of homosexuality" or the "acceptability of homosexuality as a pretended family relationship" by local authorities and schools – was indicative of the widespread homophobia at that time. (This profound and extensive homophobia obviously had an impact upon people of any gender who did not identify as heterosexual, not just upon gay and bi men.)

Fear of AIDS in the 1980s and early 1990s meant that bisexual men were stigmatised as being a 'bridge' population, spreading HIV from gay men to the rest of society. The mainstream media presented bisexual men as a shadowy, dangerous population, likely to damage 'innocent' women. (George, 1993, pp. 116–117). In addition, gay men marginalised bi men as being confused, scared or on the fence, in a way that had not happened before. Many lesbians thought bi women were letting the side down and betraying them – personally, politically and by 'risking their health'. These anti-bisexual prejudices still remain, especially, but by no means exclusively, among people who were young at that time.

What bisexuality means has changed very much since I started identifying that way 40-plus years ago. For instance, in the 1970s and 1980s I remember that bi people were much keener on the idea that relationships with men and women were complementary and that as a bisexual you would need to have relationships with a man and a woman contemporaneously. It appears that bi people now generally don't believe this, and it is often dismissed as one of those myths about bisexuality. But instead, I remember that in the past many (not all) bi people did hold these ideas. Things have changed, and such views are now considered unacceptable and untrue.

Probably the most radical change is around gender. While gay liberation and feminism have challenged ideas of male and female since around the turn of the century, the whole idea of who counts as 'man' and 'woman', what gender means, and whether one inevitably is or needs to be either a man or a woman, has undergone and is still undergoing a radical transformation. The way in which trans issues are conceptualised and discussed has changed hugely. The extent to which this has affected older people – cis or trans – is unclear, with little or no research being done on it. With an increasing number of people identifying as genderqueer, gender-fluid or non-binary, perhaps the whole notion of gender being key to sexual attraction will become less important. This is not yet the case, however.

Thus older people grew up experiencing these attitudes towards sexuality mentioned above which, thankfully, have less impact upon people who are younger now. We are all influenced by the society we grew up in and its attitudes. We are also affected by our experiences and the political landscape of the period when we became adults. For those who are or who have been politically active, this will have an enduring impact upon what we consider important and how we see ourselves. It also means that older people will not necessarily view bisexuality in the same way as do people of different generations. However, it is also vital to recognise that this may not be the case either. People, however old, often continue to change their opinions as a result of transformations within society at large and within their own lives. No one is immune from whatever happens in the present, whether or not we wholly agree with it, or whether it has turned out as we expected when we were young.

Bisexual communities

So what constitutes the UK bi community and what impact has it had upon the lives of bisexual people? What is or isn't the place of older bi people within it?

The 'official' or 'political' bi community began in the UK with the London bisexual group in 1981; this started out of anti-sexist men's groups and met at the gay men's club Heaven. There were many other groups around the UK in the 1980s and 1990s. Most of them wound up in the early 2000s, although a few remain. These groups were mainly discussion groups and they were extremely important to the people who visited them, especially as they were coming out.

Nowadays, there are many fewer real-world groups, nor is there a commercial bisexual scene. When it is possible to find sexual partners using dating apps, some kind of community with social media and all types of information on the internet, real-life communities may be less important. But they do still have their place: there are social Meet-Up groups in London and elsewhere, as well as occasional Bi Fests (informal fun days) and annual BiCons (bisexual national conferences). There are also international conferences and many bi groups in other parts of the world. Individuals who are loosely part of this politicised community are small in number, yet they are very important. Not everyone sees their sexuality politically or as part of a community; those of us who do tend to be in the minority. Nevertheless, bi people who are not part of this community do reap the benefits of our activism.

The bi community operates as a social support network, but it has also done huge amounts of valuable work, for instance, in promoting bi issues in lesbian and gay groups, often against an atmosphere of biphobia, writing letters to newspapers on bi issues, and political lobbying. This includes the long-running newsletter *Bi Community News*. In recent years, it also does all of these things on social media and has enabled the bi community and bisexuality to have a much more visible and widespread presence.

So who is in this bisexual community and who isn't? It is a liberal-left, progressive community, and has always included many who may be broadly termed 'counterculture'. My observation is that people who are or have been in this bi community generally share those beliefs to a greater or lesser extent. Bi people who do not tend not to be involved with it. It is also a well-educated, generally middle-class community, but who on average are earning less than their lesbian, gay or heterosexual counterparts (Barker et al., 2012). It is a place where – to a great extent – gender non-conformity is accepted and bi trans+ people are welcome. *The Bisexuality Report* mentioned that at one Bicon, 19 per cent of those attending identified as transgender or genderqueer (Barker et al., 2012, p. 30). There have been very few people of colour, and this has scarcely changed over the years, although the research and activism of Bi's of Colour is now having a visible and hopefully enduring impact (Applebee, 2015).

The UK-based bi community has very few visibly older bi people, with the majority of those involved in their thirties (Barker et al., 2012). This is less the case in the USA, where the community is far more established. I will return to this below. It seems fair to say that – like communities of all sorts – the politicised bi community attracts people who are like those already within it; if no one "like you" is there, you may not feel it is the place for you.

However, this political bi community is just one community where many bi people meet. It has a significant overlap with the wider queer community, an umbrella label that covers people who challenge norms of gender, sexuality or sexual behaviour in some way, and includes many individuals who are sexually attracted to, or have relationships with, people of more than one gender. Some in this queer community identify specifically as pansexual instead of bisexual, because they believe bisexuality only means 'men' and 'women' – a definition with which the bi community generally disagrees.

Many bi people also identify as polyamorous, meaning that they are – in theory and/or in practice – open to sex and emotional relationships/partnerships with more than one person. Other communities where there are many bi people are those connected specifically to sexual behaviour. These include swingers (who for the purposes of this chapter I define as people in other gender partnerships who have casual sex outside of that), and what is now referred to as the kink community – fetish clubs, BDSM, etc. There is some cross-over between those communities, and individuals who identify as bisexual or queer (George, 2003)

Identifying as bisexual [...] and not

There are also many people who would say to themselves, or to those they were intimate with, "I am bisexual" without being involved with any of these communities. Here, I am not discussing people whose primary identity or political focus is based in the queer community, although some may identify as 'lesbian' or 'gay'.

In this section, I will consider individuals who are not – or only tangentially – connected with the politicised bi community but for whom the label *bisexual* has some relevance whether or not they accept it with any enthusiasm. This includes people who reject the importance of sexual identity, those who don't want to be called 'bisexual', some who have bisexual histories but are wary of using the label in their current lives, and those who have been described as 'bisexual' for the purpose of public health interventions.

Many of these people are what I call 'reluctant identifiers'. They call themselves bisexual in some ways, under some circumstances, sometimes sharing this information with those to whom they are close, and sometimes keeping their feelings to themselves. In small-scale research I have done over the years (e.g. George, 2003, 2011) as well as approaches made to me by people anxious to 'confess' their sexuality, this contingent identity seems common.

Some of these reluctant identifiers – especially but not exclusively men – see sexuality as purely individualistic and about sex, rather than about relationships, emotions or community. If they can find partners, they do not need a community (George, 2001, pp. 35–57). They say things like: "I am just sexual"; "I like who I like, why should I restrict myself?"; "I like a specific [sexual activity/body part] that only [one gender] can provide"; "I suppose I am bisexual if I have to call myself anything"; "I'm open-minded"; "You would want to call me bisexual but I don't see it like that". Nevertheless, they may attend social activities or clubs where there are many bi people.

Some people consider taking on any sexual label to be unduly constricting, fixing an identity they consider open and flexible. They see themselves as bohemians, outsiders or artists, and view their sexuality as simply to do with the individuals concerned (Arcade, 2015).

However, there are other, specific reasons why individuals actively (or through lack of relevance or interest) reject any bi community. While the bi community is clear that people can identify as bi whatever their relationship status or experience, many bi people have trouble believing this. They consider that, because they are primarily interested in one gender, they don't have the 'right' to call themselves bisexual. Or, they don't feel they have the 'right' to identify as bi when they haven't had sex with more than one gender or anyone at all within a certain timeframe (see e.g. Bisexual.org, 2016).

Many people do identify with whomever they are partnered with, and see a bisexual identity as something that is only relevant if they are seeking a partner. Their identities may change, dependant on these relationships. Or they may consider that relationship too important to risk hurting their partner (George, 2002). Many others have a history of relationships with more than one gender but they have a very established life in communities where a bi identity would put them outside of it. This may include many communities from separatist lesbian, to orthodox religious, to close-knit extended families.

There are also 'behavioural bisexuals', often called 'men who have sex with men'. Occasionally, these terms have also been adapted for women. These labels grew out of the public health campaigns of the 1990s. These were men who had sex with men and women (with no mention of trans people then) within a certain timeframe – usually one or five years. HIV prevention programmes, unlike the bi community, were not interested in how one identified, only what one did sexually, and how safe it was (Weatherburn and Reid, 1996).

For different people, an important alliance with another community takes precedence. People who have long-standing involvement with a lesbian or gay community may, for instance, remain politically committed to that and sideline their other sexual and romantic relationships and interests. Or they may ally themselves with class politics and consider sexual identity as primarily a side issue or distraction (George, 2002). Their wider political activism is much more important to them.

Some Black and Minority Ethnic (BME) people, or people of colour, may identify primarily with those communities regardless of sexuality, with anti-racist politics, or a community specifically for Black Queers. They may experience the bisexual or wider queer community as racist, or want to reject those identities as being irrelevant, perhaps relating to one they consider more appropriate for them (Barker et al., 2012; Applebee, 2015).

Like older people in general, older bi people may consider that sexuality is not a spectrum and that they should really be fully straight or gay, even though their relationship history has been bisexual. While the YouGov (2015) surveys show that fewer people in general believe everyone is either heterosexual or homosexual, older people are far more likely to believe that there is no middle ground (18 per cent of people aged 18 to 24, 28 per cent 40 to 59, 32 per cent 60-plus).

Older people may also believe that bisexuality is for young people, not something that applies to them. Thus, if they are no longer interested in sexual relationships, or don't feel they will ever have a sexual relationship again (even if they wanted one), or don't feel they will have another relationship with another gender, there is no point in identifying as bisexual (Jones et al., 2016).

Alternatively, they may see their relationships with men/women as too different to call them 'bisexual'. Women may see their relationships with other women as primarily friendships (Shute, 1992), whereas men are their partners; men may dismiss the sex they have with other men as 'nothing important', and with women as the focus of their emotional lives. Arguably some, perhaps particularly very old people, see sex and sexuality as a private matter which has nothing to do with outsiders (Szreter and Fisher, 2010).

I have discussed these different, multifaceted identities at length in this chapter, as they are too often glossed over in much bisexual writing, with these individuals perceived as 'hard to find'. Arguably, people who are more or less closeted about their bisexuality, whether they see it as individual expression or cannot talk about it within their particular family or community, are most in need of support from out bi people.

Issues and challenges for older bi people

Those older bi people who want to find community and a social network beyond their existing group of friends and social contacts may find it elusive. The commercial lesbian or gay scene may be unwelcoming and physically inaccessible or uncomfortable for older people; social groups such as *Meet Up* may have implied, if not stated, age limits. Although, in some parts of the UK, there are community groups for lesbians and gay men, bisexuals may be very unsure of their welcome by such groups.

Bi people needing support, or biphobia-free socialising, may not necessarily get it from these groups. This may be especially true for older women, with some older lesbian groups specifically not open to bi women. The national lesbian group *Kenric*, for instance, only accepts "women who identify as lesbian". While many groups may be accepting in theory, it is hard to know in advance whether individual lesbians within it would be particularly welcoming.

At least one group – *Opening Doors London*, which works with *Age UK* to provide information and support services for people across the LGBT communities – does explicitly welcome bi people. It also runs a monthly social group for bi people over the age of 50, developed following the seminar series which gave rise to this book. However, I know of no other such projects in the UK.

In preparing for the talk from which this chapter germinated, I carried out a casual survey of some half-dozen bi people between the ages of around 51 to 72. Obviously, given that this is such a small number of people, I knew them all, and they all identified explicitly as bisexual; they simply represent a tiny snapshot of certain issues. Several things had a big impact upon how they felt about their sexuality. Some were connected broadly to getting older, and may be experienced by people regardless of sexuality. They were: caring responsibilities, and the impact that had upon their life as a whole. This could mean looking after children, but that seemed less demanding than for those who had to look after frail parents or siblings which could mean they had no time to themselves at all that would allow them to look for partners. Issues with their own health could make them isolated or unsure about their own attractiveness or abilities as a potential partner. Those two things – their own health and the health of others – meant that other things, including sexual identity or new sexual and romantic relationships, necessarily took second place.

Another significant issue was often isolation, as mentioned at the start of this section. They only socialised with people they already knew, which – if they would have liked to be in a relationship – meant that they didn't meet anyone with whom they could form relationships. Alternatively, they only met new people who were much younger, and both them, and the younger people, ruled each other out as potential partners.

Both women and men (there were no trans people within this group) remarked that they felt less confident about their sexual attractiveness and desirability as a partner than in the past. This was particularly the case for those who had experienced significant levels of ill-health.

Other issues were more directly connected to the intersections of ageing and bisexuality. For instance, I would argue that older bi people may be seen as stereotyped as hypersexual because of the connection so many make between bisexuality and sex. Given that people of colour of all ages are also often considered hypersexual, this may be particularly marked for older bi people of colour. Some respondents felt uncomfortable around younger adults as a result.

For people who were in a long-term relationship, though (and the people I talked to all identified as bi, and were out as bi to their partners – many of them long-term partners), they observed that their bisexuality had an impact upon their relationship over the very long term, but they actually found it hard to pin down what that was. If they were bi and their partner (only one of the people I talked to had significant poly relationships at that time) wasn't, then they felt there was a part of their lives that they couldn't share with them, and that did have some kind of impact.

Several remarked that they still had to come out all the time, that there were assumptions about their sexuality which were always that they were either straight or lesbian/gay. For some, this coming out had to do with ensuring that new people they met (or indeed, in advance of meeting them) knew they identified as bisexual and that this was a significant part of their lives.

Indeed, for those people who were in couples, especially long-term committed couples whether of the same or other genders, the bi-invisibility as they were getting older was very striking and this is what I have experienced myself. You are perceived as being the identity that matches the gender of your partner. If this relationship is publicly monogamous, and has lasted for many years, this conflation of partner gender and sexuality may be very difficult to break.

Gender differences in ageing

According to the longitudinal survey 'Sexual health and wellbeing among older men and women in England' (Lee et al., 2016), many people are having sex well into old age, and plentiful sexual activity is considered part of "officially sanctioned discourses of ageing well" for heterosexual couples (Segal, 2013). Much information is available online about male erectile dysfunction, with sex for older women (in committed relationships with men) concentrating on ways of rectifying their 'declining libidos'. The positive benefits of sexual activity are only stressed for people in committed couples; otherwise, it is all to do with STIs, or – in the media – women's hopeless search for a suitable partner. All other types of people in all other circumstances seem invisible, and that includes older bisexual people.

While more than half of men over the age of 70 were still sexually active in the study above, the situation around sex for older women is far more nuanced. The anecdotal indications – for instance, as mentioned by Lynne Segal in *Out of Time: The Pleasures and Perils of Ageing* (2013) – are that for some women – although by no means all – the post-menopause period signals a change in levels of interest towards sex and sexual relationships. That does not mean no interest, but rather a blunting of interest, a decrease in urgency. While this may prove a challenge for some women in existing relationships (and their partners), need this necessarily be as difficult for women who are single? The situation is unclear.

When I was researching *Bisexuality Today* in 2001/2002, I found it very difficult to track down women over the age of 50 who identified as bi. Lu was one. Aged 56 in 2002, she described her situation as follows:

> I was obsessed with being in a relationship, particularly with a man, until four or five years ago. Then I went through the menopause – quickly and easily – came out the other side and thought 'this is different'. I ended the relationship I was in and had a naturally occurring relationship with a woman. It was more intense and one-sided (from her) than I wanted. Since then I haven't been looking and no one's looking at me. So I think it's a combination of being post-menopausal and weariness of relationships.
>
> (George, 2003)

Lu's quote gives some clue as to why I may have had these difficulties. However, I can only speculate that another reason may be that women who were born before 1950 were (in 2001/2002) even more reluctant to identify as bi, due to the reasons set out earlier in this chapter. I had, however, no problem in finding bi men. They did not mention their age, except insofar as they wanted to "catch up for lost time" (George, 2003).

In *Out of Time,* Segal writes about her shame of being left by her younger male partner, and feeling humiliated that she might experience desire that is not reciprocated. On the other hand, she grudgingly accepts that some of her friends feel differently about relationships as they have grown older.

> I have little problem agreeing, at least partially, that we may desire somewhat differently, maybe even less urgently, as we dwell in old age, especially if the focus is purely on genital penetration, with all its symbolic excess. This could be why many older women, including some of my own friends, insist that they feel a new freedom now from the turbulent sexual desires of their youth.
>
> (Segal, 2013, p. 272)

Ageing for women seems more significant than it does for men. Post-menopausal women are presented as sexless and pathetic in the media. But while older men may not be considered desirable in, for instance, much of the gay scene, ageing for men does not seem to be considered a 'tragedy' in the same way that it is for women.

After her painful break-up with a man, Segal did find a new relationship – with another woman.

[Like] [...] a few other women have found in old age, they have not only been able to love again, but to love differently, experiencing, as I have, new sources of erotic pleasure and satisfaction.

(Segal, 2013, p. 269)

It seems to be an open secret that some women who had not previously been in relationships with other woman do so at this time. Why this happens, and how the women involved feel about it, seems remarkably under-researched.

Challenging the invisibility of older bi people

While in the 1980s and 1990s bisexuals seemed wholly invisible outside of the bi community, this is no longer necessarily the case. However, older bi people seem to be as invisible as ever and this is something also reported by my older bi survey group (see above). Narratives of healthy ageing aside, older people are generally not seen as sexual, and certainly not as bisexual. Sometimes older bi men can be seen as bi in a very negative way by both women and men – predatory, unattractive, undesirable. Older women are generally seen as invisible whatever their sexuality. If by some fluke it is certain that they are sexual, then they become Dirty Old Women – cougars, MILFS, predators. Given that a key stereotype of bi women is that we are promiscuous, it is possible that older bi women are considered hypersexual in a way that other women are not.

When I have experienced contempt or disgust for my bisexual identity in recent years, it has been from much younger people who do not want to think that older people are actively sexual (as that is how they see it) and particularly not with more than one gender. Conversely, some younger people seem encouraged that sex need not stop for them however old they are.

So what does this enduring invisibility mean? Where are the older bisexuals now? It seems the case that – in the face of potential contempt – most older bi people are not out in most circumstances. Those older people who do unequivocally identify as bisexual – for instance, those who have been part of long-standing bi communities – may have experienced very significant levels of biphobia when they were younger. They have found acceptance within their friendship network and moved away from activism because being out all the time can be pretty exhausting.

As we have seen above, what bisexuality means changes over time, and the way an individual relates to their bisexuality also relates to where they are in their lifespan. In addition, the way bisexuality is viewed by society changes over time. We are all influenced by the times, and socio-political climate, in which we grew up, as well as changing and growing in the here and now. Thus all of those combined *may* mean that older bi people see their bisexuality very differently to younger generations, and they may not connect to the current bi community. These generation gaps are tendencies or generalisations rather than hard-and-fast rules, but they do apply to some or to many.

Social media can be extremely helpful in allowing you to express and be at ease with your bisexuality, and to experience a type of visibility. But what happens if older people do not use social media, either because they do not have access to it, or because they actively or pre-emptively reject it (as being only for the young, or a potentially hostile, privacy-invading waste of time)?

Much of the activism, research and other work that has been done around older people and bisexuality is from the USA, where the bi community is more established than in the UK. However, their social, political and cultural references are different from those we experience here and so any exact correlation needs to be treated with caution. For instance, the fundamentalist Christian and moral right has little influence in the UK; in the USA, there is next to no welfare state, so an individual may feel compelled to stay in a job or marriage where their sexuality must stay hidden, rather than lose the medical benefits they gain through it. Identity labels of all types also seem more readily adopted in the USA, including those for older people such as boomers, seniors or elders.

Nevertheless, this activism in the USA is exciting and useful for people in the UK. For instance, the series of YouTube videos called #StillBisexual features people (of a wide age range, including over 70) using a range of text-based posters indicating they are counteracting clichés about bisexuality by being 'still bisexual'. The Bi Elders Facebook group shares information and offers informal support. Some of these Bi Elders include people who have been bi activists for decades, and met President Obama to lobby for bi rights.

At the end of 2013, I 'email interviewed' six bi people over the age of 50 for my blog *Bisexuality and Beyond* who responded to requests on the blog, through personal contacts and through social media. I did not require that they be willing to post photographs of themselves (they could use any illustration) or use their real names. Given the great lack of visible older bi people, I am very pleased that this was successful. However, those who responded were all very out and were in no way indicative of the vast range of people for whom the label 'bisexual' might be relevant. It proved too difficult to find people who weren't white, from the USA and mostly with an activist background. As a result, this interview project is currently on hold. The need for a wider variety of older bi people willing to be visible remains.

It seems very likely that such a high level of invisibility leads to isolation which can lead, in turn, to poor mental health. A growing body of research indicates that bi people have lower levels of mental health than do lesbians or gay men, who in turn have worse mental health than do heterosexuals (Barker et al., 2012). An analysis of the bi women's responses in the 2007 Stonewall Women's Health Survey showed that the bi respondents may be more likely to experience social stress due to the 'double discrimination' of homophobia and biphobia. While bi respondents were more likely to be young than the lesbian cohort, older bi women were more likely to have suicidal thoughts (Colledge et al., 2015).

This connects very closely to the reasons why considering bisexuality and ageing is so important, and why research on it – along with additional intersections such as race, class, poverty, disability – is key. This is particularly true regarding loneliness and isolation.

If you are isolated, you cannot ask for support when you need it. Important parts of your life may be unknown to, or rejected by, people to whom you are close and, as you grow older, to people caring for you. You may feel the lack of other people like you, without really knowing who they are or where they are. Perhaps with less isolation and invisibility, older bi people might be better able to capitalise on what the older bisexuals I contacted also said: that bisexuality had been very positive for them, far more so than this chapter may indicate. They considered they had lived authentically, even as they wished things had been easier.

While much of this chapter has been about the disadvantages or difficulties of being an older bi person, there are also many advantages to ageing for bi people. For instance, older people may care less about what others think. Other people may find it more difficult to say you will change your mind or will inevitably 'settle down'. The feeling that time is running out may impel us to act on our feelings rather than pushing them away. It can also be encouraging for younger people to see that they have 'elders' and that people before them have experienced similar challenges and overcome them.

Conclusion and suggestions for further work

This chapter is entitled "You're not *still* bisexual, are you?" because this is something that has often been said to me in recent years. Of course, I am still bisexual and this remains a very positive part of my life. While mainstream society may find this hard to understand, and some lesbian and gay people remain unconvinced, even now, my sexual identity has clearly stayed with me!

Now that I have identified as bisexual for more than 40 years, and have spent 30-plus years in and around the British bi community, I wonder what all the other bisexuals I have met over that time are doing now. For sure, not all of them still identify as bi but what about those many who do? How can this invisibility be challenged? What research needs to be done and by whom? What do older bisexuals want? A first step would be to ask us.

There is so much scope for further research, as well as for further political activism. Intrinsic to all of this, there has to be a recognition that bi people encompass a wide variety of individuals across every possible intersection, and of life experience already lived and to come. All research should be carried out with the explicit involvement of older bi people ourselves. I conclude this chapter with some suggestions.

Older bi people and the bisexual community

Research should be done to see how the bi community and older bi people could connect more effectively, along with considering how a wider range of older bi people see their sexuality.

Intergenerational projects

One of the issues across the wider queer community seems to be a division between older and younger people. Intergenerational projects could be developed by older and younger people together, specifically to address this issue. This should take place outside of any commercial 'scene'.

Coming out later in life

One of the major differences between older bi people seems to be between those who have been out for much of their lives and those who come out later. While it is hard to come out as bi at any time in one's life, coming out in much later life surely requires an enormous amount of bravery and effort, risking rejection and possibly great financial difficulties or loss. There are people who have identified in one way for most of their lives, perhaps without considering any other options, and then – after the end of a relationship – they become attracted to someone of another gender. What should they call themselves? What sort of bi community do they need, and how could it be developed? How can other bi people support them, if this is what they want?

Old age

The issues for bi people in much older age, or with dementia, or significant ill-health, remain unclear. What about partners and families who don't know about significant areas of their loved ones' lives, for instance, or who disapprove of those things? Or recognition and support by health and social care professionals of those people closest to us, whether or not our blood relatives are supportive of this? What about women with mainly lesbian lives who have support from a family of choice – and whose chosen family rejects bisexuality? Much more research is needed here.

References

Applebee, J. (2015) Bis of colour survey report. https://bisexualresearch.files.wordpress.com/2015/06/bis-of-colour-survey-report.pdf (accessed 30 December 2015).

Arcade, P. (2015) Penny Arcade remembers Holly Woodlawn. *Out* Magazine. www. out.com/entertainment/2015/12/10/penny-arcade-remembers-holly-woodlawn (accessed 30 December 2015).

Barker, M., Richards, C., Jones, R., Bowes-Catton, H., Plowman, T., Yockney, J. and Morgan, M. (2012). *The Bisexuality Report: Bisexual Inclusion in LGBT Equality and Diversity.* Milton Keynes: The Open University Centre for Citizenship, Identities and Governance.

Bisexual.org (2016) *This Bi Life: I Don't Feel Bi Enough.* https://bisexual.org/this-bi-life-i-dont-feel-bi-enough/ (accessed 22 October 2017).

Bisexual Resource Center (n.d.) *Way Beyond the Binary.* www.biresource.net/waybeyondthebinary.shtml (accessed 30 December 2015).

Clarke, V. (2008) *From Outsiders to Motherhood to Reinventing the Family: Constructions of Lesbians Parenting in the Psychological Literature – 1886–2006.* University of the West of England, E-pub (accessed 29 January 2016).

Colledge, L. (2015) 'Poorer mental health in UK bisexual women than lesbians: Evidence from the UK 2007 Stonewall Women's Health Survey', *Journal of Public Health,* 37(3): 427–437.

Diamond, L. (2008) *Sexual Fluidity: Understanding Women's Love and Desire.* Cambridge, MA: Harvard University Press.

George, S. (1993) *Women and Bisexuality.* London: Scarlet Press.

George, S. (2001) 'Making sense of bisexual personal ads', *Journal of Bisexuality,* 1(4): 35–57.

George, S. (2002) 'British bisexual women: A new century', *Journal of Bisexuality,* 2(2–3): 175–191.

George, S. (2003) *Bisexuality Today.* Unpublished manuscript.

George, S. (2006–2016) *Bisexuality and Beyond* blog (bisexualityandbeyond.com).

George, S. (2011) 'Ten years after: How the internet has changed everything and British bi women', *Journal of Bisexuality,* 11(4): 426–433.

Houlbrook, M. (2005) *Queer London: Perils and Pleasures in the Sexual Metropolis 1918–57.* Chicago, IL: University of Chicago Press.

Jones, RL., Almack, K. and Scicluna, R. (2016) *Ageing and Bisexuality: Case Studies from 'The Looking Both Ways' Project.* Milton Keynes: The Open University.

Lee, DM., Nazroo, J., O'Connor, DB., Blake, M. and Pendleton, N. (2016) 'Sexual health and wellbeing among older men and women in England', *Archives of Sexual Behavior,* 45(1): 133–144.

Ochs, R. (2016) *A Few Quotes from Robyn Ochs.* http://robynochs.com/bisexual/ (accessed 25 January 2016).

Porter, K. and Weeks, J. (1990) *Between the Acts: Lives of Homosexual Men 1885–1967.* London: Routledge.

Power, L. (1995) *No Bath but Plenty of Bubbles: Stories from the Gay Liberation Front 1970–73.* London: Continuum.

Segal, L. (2013) *Out of Time: The Pleasures and Perils of Ageing.* London: Verso Books.

Shute, N. (1931) *Another Man's Poison.* London: Robert Hale.

Shute, N. (1992) *Passionate Friends.* London: Robert Hale.

Still bisexual website. http://stillbisexual.com/category/bisexual-elders/ (accessed 25 January 2016).

Szreter, S. and Fisher, K. (2010) *Sex before the Sexual Revolution: Intimate Life in England 1918–63.* Cambridge: Cambridge University Press.

Weatherburn, P. and Reid, D. (1996) *Behaviourally Bisexual Men in the UK: Another Population to Prioritise?* London: the HIV Project.

Wolff, C. (1971) *Love between Women*. London: Quartet.

Wolff, C. (1977) *Bisexuality: A Study*. London: Quartet.

YouGov (2015) '1 in 2 young people say they are not 100% heterosexual'. https://yougov.co.uk/news/2015/08/16/half-young-not-heterosexual/ (accessed 5 January 2016).

YouGov US (2015) 'A third of young Americans say they aren't 100% heterosexual'. https://today.yougov.com/news/2015/08/20/third-young-americans-exclusively-heterosexual/ (accessed 5 January 2016).

4 Mental health and well-being among older trans people

Louis Bailey, Jay McNeil and Sonja J. Ellis

Introduction

Trans[1] ageing is a much neglected area of knowledge within the field of LGBT ageing (Fredriksen-Goldsen et al., 2014), and the mental health and well-being of older trans people even more so. This chapter presents findings from the Trans Mental Health Study (McNeil et al., 2012) as they relate to the mental health of trans people who are 50 years of age and older and living in the UK. The Trans Mental Health Study (TMHS) was the first comprehensive study of trans people's experiences of mental health and well-being, and remains the largest British survey of trans people to date. Research focused on how being trans impacts upon people's mental health in the course of their everyday lives, as well as the role played by social/medical gender transition on mental health and well-being. While 889 respondents completed the survey, the analysis used in this chapter is based on the answers of 127 respondents who were older than 50 years of age at the time the survey was completed (2012). The chapter first discusses the small but growing body of literature about trans ageing and mental health. Second, the chapter briefly discusses the methodology of the TMHS before exploring two key areas: first, how older trans adults rated their mental health and well-being and the role of being trans in that assessment; second, the role of mental health services and informal sources of support on older trans people's mental health later in life. The chapter concludes with a number of suggestions and recommendations for further research and policy/practice initiatives.

Trans ageing and mental health

There is a growing body of literature around both trans ageing and the mental health of older trans adults, although the vast majority of this literature is not from the UK. While it is a good thing that this knowledge gap is being addressed, we do need to know more at a global level about trans people's experiences of ageing and older trans people's mental health. Furthermore, a gap remains in UK-based research to understand in greater depth the mental health experiences of older trans people in the UK and, more significantly, the complex ways in which mental health is interrelated to trans ageing.

It is clear from some of the existing non-UK-based surveys that older trans people are more at risk of depressive symptomology and, to an extent, anxiety than are their cisgender peers (Fredriksen-Goldsen et al., 2014; Riggs et al., 2015). However, this broad statement does obscure issues around if and when a person transitions (earlier in life, during later life, or not at all), the stage of life they currently occupy, their generation and the extent of connectedness to family, friends and support services, both formal and informal.

The THMS main study, alongside others, suggests that trans people's mental health improves following transition (McNeil et al., 2012). Riggs et al. (2015), summarising studies of trans people's mental health, well-being and needs in Australia, provide evidence to suggest that older trans people have better mental health than do younger trans people. Further studies have also demonstrated that older trans people have higher levels of resilience later in life and therefore, to quote Tarryn Witten, 'it's not all darkness' (Witten, 2014, p. 24). Meanwhile, other studies indicate that trans women have poorer psychological well-being than trans men or those who identify as non-binary (Warren et al., 2016).

The aforementioned studies do not downplay the ongoing and detrimental effects of cisgenderism across the life course: 'the ideology that invalidates people's own understanding of their genders and bodies' (Ansara, 2015, p. 14). Indeed, as Bailey (2012) has argued elsewhere, a life course approach to trans people's well-being, which recognises the effects of discrimination, violence, harassment across people's lives, is important. While Pearce (Chapter 5, this volume), points to the importance of challenging normative notions of ageing and the life course with respect to trans people's life experiences, it remains important to assess life course factors when assessing older trans people's mental health and well-being.

Overall, when considering the mental health of older trans people, there is a need to understand the complexity of mental health experiences among older trans adults and to move beyond rather one-dimensional approaches which equate trans ageing to poor mental health. In addition, this is important not only to fill existing knowledge gaps, especially in the UK, but also to ensure that mental health and older people's services can better serve their older trans clients.

Methods

The TMHS was conducted online and comprised a series of fixed response and open response questions, as well as standardized tests. The final dataset comprised 889 respondents. The data drawn on in the remainder of this chapter relate to 127 respondents aged 50 years and older. Content analysis (Green and Thorogood, 2004) was applied to the qualitative sections of the data and a critical realist approach has been taken whereby respondents have been treated as key informants about their experiences. As such, data relating to open-ended questions rely on self-reporting. All relevant qualitative data presented here have been analysed inductively, and Nvivo has been used to code and identify recurrent themes (Green and Thorogood, 2004). These themes have then been used to expand on and account for any significant patterns raised by the quantitative data.

Sample characteristics

Identity labels included the following: trans man, trans woman, man with a transsexual history, woman with a transsexual history, androgyne, bigender, gender neutral, neutrois, genderqueer, non-gendered, non-binary, Kathoey (a Thai term for trans women), Khusra (a Punjabi term for trans), cross-dresser, transvestite, transgender person. In terms of constancy or otherwise of gender identity, 27 per cent of the sample had a constant and clear identity as a man; 38 per cent had a constant and clear identity as a woman; 4 per cent had a constant and clear non-binary identity; 23 per cent had a variable or fluid non-binary identity; 3 per cent had no gender identity, and 5 per cent were 'unsure'. The ages of respondents ranged from 50 to 75 years. In terms of ethnicity, 96.8 per cent of respondents were White British/ Welsh/Scottish/English/Irish/Northern Irish, the remainder being non-White British (British Chinese or other mixed/multiple ethnic background).

Older trans people's mental health and well-being

Baseline mental health

A total of 123 participants rated their mental health using a 7-point scale whereby 1 represented 'very poor' and 7 represented 'excellent'. Twenty-six per cent of respondents rated their mental health at 7 (excellent), while 8 per cent rated it at 1 (very poor). The mean score was 4.98, as compared to 3.7 for the general TMHS sample (n=565), showing that, overall, older trans participants felt that their mental health was fairly good. In terms of mental health issues and concerns, 56 participants gave details. Of those with a current diagnosis (n=34) the most common diagnoses were depression (n=10), anxiety (n=8) and stress (n=8). Twenty-one participants had been diagnosed with difficulties in the past but no longer retained these diagnoses. Again, depression was the most common (n=15), followed by stress (n=9) and anxiety (n=8). These figures reflect the findings of other studies of the prevalence of depressive symptomatology among older trans adults (Fredriksen-Goldsen et al., 2014).

Impact of being trans upon mental health

Respondents were asked whether being trans or having a trans history affected their mental health. The majority of respondents (41%) felt that being trans had a mixed impact upon their overall mental health. Two respondents who had transitioned discussed the varied impact of this upon their mental health:

> I feel better internally but am also aware that many parts of society will not understand/accept what I am.

> Having transitioned has made me much happier, but also subjected me to discrimination.

Thus, counter to assumptions that mental health improves post-transition for trans people, the above quotes indicate that this is sometimes qualified by ongoing accounts of what may be termed 'minority stress' (Hendricks and Testa, 2012). Actual or anticipated experiences of rejection and other forms of discrimination have been identified as a salient internal stressor for trans individuals, with associated impacts upon well-being (Rood et al., 2016).

For the 16 per cent who felt that being trans or having a trans history positively affected their mental health, the counter position relates to affirming ideas of resilience suggested by Witten (2014) who identifies the positive affect of coming to terms with one's gender identity or expression. These respondents answered thus:

> All my depression was caused by suppressing my true self.

> Cross-dressing gives me a feeling of well-being and allows me to express my feminine side.

The remaining respondents (28%) were either not sure or felt that this correlation had no relevance to their experience.

The significance of both the life course and generational differences may be seen in the following comment:

> I see these youngsters not having the problems those of my era seemed to have, and I feel jealous. Can't help it even though I know it is silly and wrong to feel this way.

Interestingly, one respondent who stated that being trans had no impact upon their mental health explained that they were fortunate in being able to have the space to deal with their gender issues during childhood, again illustrating the significance of a life course perspective:

> I was lucky enough to be allowed considerable latitude in gender expression during childhood – which for the 1960s/1970s was exceptional I know [...] but as a result I have had very little resentment or anger/confusion over being trans.

The comments of the respondents who felt that being trans had a negative impact upon their mental health (15%) are particularly illuminating and reveal a deep-rooted sense of shame and guilt about their identity:

> I feel I am a burden to everyone. [...] I wish I was dead a lot of the time [...] I wish I had not been born all mixed up.

> The damage done to me as a trans person of 30 years of repressed and internalised shame, guilt, fear, etc. is incalculable. So many of us are twisted, stunted caricatures of the people we might have been.

The survey also explored what trans people pre-transition felt could improve their mental health. Nineteen respondents felt that transition would help in terms of alleviating symptoms of gender dysphoria and bringing their bodies in line with their felt sense of gendered self ('Being seen by the GIC [Gender Identity Clinic] and having an acceptable outcome that allows me to match my body to my mind'). Others wanted clarity about their gender, having someone to talk to, receiving support, being acknowledged by others for who they are and having more confidence with regard to social life. Five respondents cited that having a society that was more understanding and accepting of trans issues would serve to improve their mental health.

Self-esteem

A total of 124 participants completed a 7-point Likert scale rating of self-esteem, from very low (1) to very high (7). Thirty-one per cent rated their self-esteem as fairly high (6), 16 per cent as very high (7), while 13 per cent rated it very low (1). The mean score was 4.45, which is slightly higher than the mean score for the whole THMS sample: 3.7.

Approximately one-third of respondents felt that being trans had a positive effect on their self-esteem. The respondents who expanded on why this was so emphasised that they felt 'proud' to be trans, or highlighted the skills or virtues it had given them:

> I now consider myself gender gifted.

Elsewhere, respondents felt that the changes they had made had been positive:

> I have extra confidence compared to before I 'came out'.

> I understand myself more now than I ever have.

> Since I transitioned I have never felt better. It's the best thing I've ever done.

The 13 per cent who felt that being trans had a negative effect on their self-esteem cited the following as factors: feeling that they were not able to be themselves; feeling that being trans was, in itself, negative; feeling disconnected from the social world and experiencing rejection from family members and friends. The following quote highlights the last two factors:

> I don't feel as though I am included in my family's life or plans, nor do I feel included socially by either the men or women at work.

For the respondents who felt mixed, this was either because their perceptions had changed over the course of their transition due to a differing relationship to one's self, as the following quote demonstrates:

> Sometimes you feel good about yourself because you know you are now in a body that goes some way to agree with how your mind sees yourself, other times you think your body isn't as good as you want it to be.

Or this was due to the discrepancy between having a positive relationship to one's self versus negative experiences at a societal level, as the following quotes reveal:

> I'm much happier with myself since I transitioned, but it has also caused others to think much less of me.

> I enjoy the change of role when cross-dressed, but find it scary to go out in the street or to pubs or restaurants dressed.

Interestingly, when compared to the general sample, this demographic of older trans people had a significantly more positive interpretation of being trans when it came to self-esteem, again highlighting the significance of resilience. This finding is also reflected in Australian studies, as highlighted by Riggs et al. (2015). While only 18 per cent of the general sample felt that being trans positively impacted upon their self-esteem, for the older trans people the figure was 33 per cent. Similarly, 26 per cent of the general sample felt that being trans negatively impacted upon their self-esteem, compared to just 13 per cent from the older demographic.

Control over life

Respondents were asked about the amount of control they felt they had over their lives in the present moment on a scale of (1) indicating no control to (7) indicating total control. The mean score for the older trans respondents was 5, higher than that for the general sample (3.8).

Respondents were also asked to what extent being trans had impacted upon their sense of control over their entire lives. The majority of respondents (32%) felt that being trans had a mixed impact. In nearly all cases, this related to the discrepancy between feeling at peace with being trans and feeling in control with personal aspects of transition, in contrast to the lack of control they felt around other people's reactions to their gender or institutional mechanisms which govern transition:

> Positive because I understand myself and which direction I need to travel. Negative because transitioning will affect family relationships and work prospects.

> The GIC [Gender Identity Clinic] have too much control on my life and what will happen and when.

One respondent, who felt unsure, said simply:

> There are certain days when I can dress [as I want] and some when I cannot. These are fixed by my family and work routines. I accept this quite happily.

However, although the above statement suggests that this is a rule imposed upon the respondent by family members and colleagues, it is not completely clear.

Thirty per cent of respondents felt that being trans had no impact upon the amount of control they felt over their life. However, where respondents expanded upon this, it became clear that although they felt that they had control in general life, they did not feel that they had any control in relation to their transition because, in the words of this respondent:

> it's all down to gatekeepers and people in multiple NHS local health boards who really don't have a clue.

Another respondent felt that they now have control over their life, but that the time in which they transitioned – in this case during the 1970s – meant that they felt they had little control over some of the penalties that occurred as a result of their transition:

> My one regret is that, since I changed during the seventies, when one had to abandon one's career, disappear, and then start all over again, this has cost me dear in financial terms. I now live in a tiny one-bedroom flat to which I cannot even invite a visitor to call upon me, and I live on a much smaller pension income than I should have had if I had remained male.

For those who felt that being trans had a positive influence on the degree of control they had in their life (15%), this related to feeling more connected with themselves and feeling in control of their transition:

Now I accept who I am and can be myself, I have much more control over my life as I allow myself to be the person I am and I'm no longer afraid to be trans.

I feel empowered by making this step in my life. I am going to transition and nobody will stop me.

The following comments sum up the situation of those who felt that being trans impacted negatively upon the amount of control they had over their life (13%), and related to actual or perceived experiences of fallout as a result of being trans/transitioning:

Since becoming openly transgender my life and career has been dismantled through no fault of my own.

Hiding who I am means that I do not push forward for certain promotions at work in case of being found out or having to explain myself; therefore, I do not push ahead.

I do not feel able to do all that I wish to do because I am concerned about being trans and being outed as such. I feel as though I need to keep my head down, particularly at home, where I am now living alone in a new neighbourhood.

Life satisfaction

Respondents were asked about how satisfied they felt with their lives, using Diener's 'Satisfaction with Life' scale. This is a 5-item scale designed to measure global cognitive judgements of one's life satisfaction (not a measure of either positive or negative affect). Respondents indicate how much they agree or disagree with each of the 5 items using a 7-point scale that ranges from 7 strongly agree to 1 strongly disagree. The mean score was 14.14, which, interestingly, was less than the mean score for the general sample which was 19. Regret about lack of opportunities for transition over the life course, as well as the social 'fallout' of being trans, became dominant factors for the slightly reduced life satisfaction ratings.

Respondents also assessed what they felt the impact of being trans was for their life satisfaction. Fifty-one per cent reported that being trans had a mixed impact upon their life satisfaction, and one respondent said that while they were now happy with their body due to reassignment, they felt that it was still not what they wanted it to be had they 'been born physically male'.

A handful of respondents felt comfortable with who they are now, but noted that the experience of being misgendered or enduring prejudicial attitudes had negatively impacted upon their life satisfaction. For those who reported that being trans had a negative impact, the reasons either related to gender dysphoria:

> I don't like waking up every day knowing that I don't have the body parts that I am meant to have

or by not being able to live as their felt gender:

> I have chosen to live as male, considering this to be the best compromise.

In addition, respondents experienced external and sometimes extreme barriers around discrimination, harassment and waiting for gender reassignment:

> Death threats, abandonment, exclusion, financial ruin, destruction of my career.

For those who cited that being trans had a positive impact, by far the largest response related to feeling that coming to terms with being trans and transitioning (social and/or medical) had served to increase their satisfaction with their life:

> Since making the commitment to be true to myself and live in my acquired gender, I am now at peace with myself and the world around me.

While being trans had a mostly mixed impact upon life satisfaction, when specific questions about the impact of transition and 'coming out' were factored in, a different story emerged, one which was mostly positive. Sixty-three per cent of respondents reported that they felt more satisfied as a result of telling others they are trans, while only 8 per cent were less satisfied.

Those who reported feeling more satisfied cited receiving a mostly positive reception after telling family and friends that they were trans and felt that this, in turn, made them feel more comfortable in themselves:

> Coming out to friends has enabled me to be myself around them, and I no longer feel like I have to hide under a façade.

In contrast, respondents who felt less satisfied after telling others about their trans status or history cited negative reactions and falling out with family and friends as the root cause:

> My daughter was appalled. [...] My husband told me I was making a mistake.

Of the 88 respondents who had transitioned, the majority (64%) reported feeling more satisfied since transitioning. This related to feeling able to be themselves, feeling more comfortable in their bodies and feeling that their gender was recognised by others:

> I have a great deal more satisfaction with the body I now have and pride in my determination to achieve it.

> Being able to be myself at all times. Being seen by others as I really am.

One of the three respondents who felt less satisfied after transitioning explained how:

> The outcomes of my surgery and hormonal treatment have [...] been unsatisfactory [and that this] outweigh[s] the happiness that comes from living in my true/felt gender.

The other respondent who felt less satisfied described how they now have no job:

> I had no choice and now have no job and have been bullied by friends, family, work into retirement and sickness. I hate what I am and would like to just never wake up.

The third respondent did not expand on their answer.

It is clear from the data presented in this section that wider social networks and relationships have a significant impact upon older trans people's mental health and well-being. This was also explored in the TMHS in relation to formal mental health services.

Formal mental health services

Seventy-four respondents completed this section of the survey. Of those who reported having used NHS mental health services, 46 per cent were satisfied or very satisfied, while 28 per cent felt dissatisfied or very dissatisfied (n=74). In the general sample, a larger majority (63%) were satisfied/very satisfied whilst 34 per cent were dissatisfied/very dissatisfied with their experiences (n=396).

Issues reported in relation to levels of satisfaction with mental health services may be grouped into the following themes:

1   Lack of trust:

> Lack of trust after being committed in 1978.

2   Lack of access to services:

> These facilities were not available when I was changing over. Support was provided by other trans people through SHAFT.

> I can't get past the first hurdle. At my GPs you have to be very as-
> sertive, tell lies, to get *anything* let alone a referral. I'm afraid I'm a
> wimpy little mouse. My GP ridiculed me when I asked for help.

3   Lack of resources:

> Overall, I believe they are caring and trying to help people as
> best they can, but are increasingly limited by time and budgetary
> constraints.

> I live in a remote rural area and mental health services are inflexible
> and poorly funded.

4   Lack of knowledge of trans issues:

> [A]t the final session discounted my comment about having joined a tv ts
> social website as 'cross-dressing is something peculiarly English'.

> [H]e asked 'Tell me how long have you been dressing as a woman?'
> I answered 'which stereotype do you want to use?'

Respondents were also asked to what extent they had been open with mental
health professionals about their trans status. The majority of respondents
(46%) stated, 'yes, completely open', followed by 18 per cent who stated, 'yes,
sometimes', 12 per cent 'rarely' and 11 per cent of respondents 'never' disclosed their status to mental health practitioners.

Those who had experienced transphobia within mental health services
were invited to further expand on their experiences. The following statements from participants are particularly illuminating:

> They have no awareness of gender issues. [...] They have a comfort zone
> in regards to treating recognised mental health problems. I do not have
> a mental health issue, regarding being a woman. It is not a mental health
> problem. Antidepressants will not help gender identity issues!

> I was asked if I'd had a boyfriend in my life. I didn't see the point in this
> question as I was asking if I could be referred for GRS [gender reassign-
> ment surgery].

> Wrongly prescribed antipsychotic by Christian psychiatrist – I stopped
> after first dose and obtained a second (different) opinion.

Accessing mental health services in the future

A clear majority of respondents (72%) would access mental health services
in the future if they needed to, 20 per cent were unsure, while 8 per cent
would not (n=127). Respondents were then asked whether they had any concerns about accessing mental health services in the future because of their

trans status/history. The majority (63%) did not have any concerns, while 24 per cent of respondents did have concerns. A further 13 per cent were unsure. These figures are in keeping with the results from the general sample, with 74 per cent who would access mental health services in the future and 50 per cent who did not have any concerns.

Some respondents who would access mental health services in the future highlighted the importance of attending as a means of highlighting the existence and needs of trans people:

> I think they need to be exposed to trans people to address these issues.

> If they don't know that certain types of needs from patients (and certain types of patients exist in the first place), the need will never be addressed.

In keeping with this, respondents who would not access mental health services in the future expressed distrust that they would be treated with dignity and their needs respected:

> Coming out has marked my copy book. I do worry that some mental health professionals believe we trans people are delusional.

> I would be concerned that some ignorant and prejudiced idiots might (even after 30 years) still try to link any difficulty back to the fact that 30 years ago I had SRS.

For some, this was based on previous bad experience:

> I was forced to see one as a 13-year-old. Am psychologostic phobic.

> Very bad experience previously makes me not want to risk a repeat.

Other respondents felt unsure:

> What reception can I expect?

Seeking help when distressed

In response to the question 'Have you ever felt so distressed that you needed to seek help or support urgently?', 60 respondents said 'yes', 64 said 'no', and 3 were unsure (n=127). Of particular concern is the follow-on finding that, when asked if they have ever avoided urgent help or support when distressed because of being trans, 27 respondents stated 'yes' and 33 stated 'no' (n=63). Respondents were then invited to expand on their answers with comments:

> Lack of trust due to history with mental institutions/workers [this respondent had been sectioned for being trans – declared in previous answers].

You bottle it up, you force it down and try to cope yourself because the fear of society's reaction, the stigma and shame is so powerful you would rather die or go mad than reveal your trans-ness.

I avoided help before 'coming out', as I wanted to hide things. Now, I will ask if I need [help].

At the root of these responses are fears of being pathologised as well as actual experiences across the life course of negative encounters with health and social care staff and services whereby respondents felt ridiculed on account of their trans status, representative of the trickle-down effect of negative portrayals of transgenderism in wider society.

Participants were asked about the sources they turned to when they needed urgent help or support. Their general practitioner (GP) was the most popular (24 responses), followed by a LGBT helpline (19) and trans friends (17). Building on this, respondents were then asked what forms of support they found to be helpful in a crisis. By far the majority of respondents cited trans-specific support, both in terms of formal support (such as trans social/support groups or online trans resources) or informal support (via trans friends):

I got help within the TG community – nobody else ever helped.

Trans friends were helpful, because they understood what I was talking about.

I first sought help in about 1971 when I had my first suicide attempt as I just could not carry on any more – that scared me so much that I telephoned the Manchester Gay Switchboard and spoke to a very caring young woman, who listened to my thoughts and feelings without judgement. She was the first person I ever revealed my trans nature to and she was very helpful.

In contrast, when asked about which sources of support they found to be unhelpful in a crisis, some respondents cited instances of NHS staff ignorance and negative attitudes, which they found offputting. Respondents cited instances of being misgendered, both in person and over the phone, when requesting help, and bemoaned the patronising attitudes of some medical professionals.

One respondent cited an instance of a GP who left them feeling suicidal and that, as a result, they 'decided to go it alone'. Another respondent noted 'a lack of understanding and ridicule' when they initially sought help. In both this and the previous case, however, the exact circumstances were not revealed. Other particularly worrying accounts were cited:

I have often been told that "we cannot help people like you".

A Sister in A&E had a problem with me being trans or lesbian, not sure which. I was left in agony for far too long without being seen.

Some respondents cited a lack of consistency in front-line training, especially around dignity and respect, as well as a general lack of knowledge about trans issues by NHS staff. One respondent cited instances in which their trans identity was pathologised:

> People would always assume sexual abuse is the cause and they would keep relating to something that never happened.

It is clear from this section of the chapter that formal mental health services were problematic for many of the respondents in some way or another. First, there was a sense in which these services were necessary but not always accessible. Second, some respondents identified issues of poor practice and discrimination. In light of this, respondents also spoke about other sources of support that they may, or may not, turn to in order to support their mental well-being. Respondents found friends, especially trans friends, to be by far the most supportive of respondents' gender identity. Relationships with a spouse/partner and family members (such as parents and siblings) were more mixed, being dependent on unique family dynamics and intensely personal reactions to news of gender transition.

Some respondents recounted instances of their children initially being 'shocked and unhappy', 'difficult' or 'hostile', but stated that family members had since adjusted to the change and were now 'supportive'. One respondent revealed that their children did not know while another said that their children had overlooked it 'as a phase'. Some respondents had mixed experiences within their families, with some of their children being more accepting than their other children. One respondent described how they had left their children because they wanted to 'protect them from abuse', while another respondent revealed that their son did experience bullying at school because of their parent's trans status. Some respondents reported how, since transition, their children were no longer in contact. In a few cases, this extended to grandchildren as well:

> My daughter and son-in-law decided to stop me seeing my granddaughters and therefore I do not have contact with them either.

One respondent described how they lost custody of their children following their transition:

> My wife forced the sale of our marital home in January 2012 and my two daughters went with her as she had bought a three-bedroom home by the time I found out what was happening. I was only able to find a one-bedroom home in the time available.

Another respondent described how they had raised a child with a previous partner but had no parental rights once the relationship ended.

Conclusion

This chapter has demonstrated that older trans people reported better rates of mental health compared to the general sample, in addition to higher rates of self-esteem and control over their lives. This accords with research found in other countries, particularly the suggestion that older trans people report better mental health than young trans people (Riggs et al., 2015). However, it was apparent from the THMS that older trans people's life satisfaction was lower. Although there was a marked improvement in life satisfaction as a result of 'coming out' and transitioning, the lower life satisfaction rates were, in large part, due to regrets about not being able to transition earlier on in the life course. Respondents cited the loss they felt about not being able to transition at a younger age, detailing their frustrations about growing up during a time when understanding and awareness of transgenderism was lacking. As a result, respondents missed out on particularly formative gendered experiences during childhood and adolescence. In addition, not transitioning earlier meant that the symptoms of gender dysphoria were prolonged, which may have had ramifications for mental health, confidence and opportunities, and overall quality of life over the life course. This accords with the findings of the wider sample of the THMS (McNeil et al., 2012) that mental health improves post-transition. However, being forced to transition later on in life meant that respondents will have to navigate hormones and surgery via an ageing body, which can result in complications and less satisfactory outcomes (Bailey, 2012). However, an argument can be made for putting off certain surgeries until medical advancements have caught up with demand and improved the surgical techniques available (Bailey, 2012).

The majority of respondents had a positive relationship to their trans identity, highlighting the protective qualities of a secure internal sense of self. However, where being trans or transitioning had a negative impact upon their mental health, in nearly all cases this was related to external factors linked to societal transphobia and associated stigma which filtered down to the workplace, the street and personal relationships, creating minority stress which, when spread over the life course, can be particularly damaging as the result of a cumulative effect.

Where respondents felt dissatisfied with mental health services (28%), this was mainly in relation to previous negative experiences and encountering a lack of awareness of trans issues. One person was sectioned for being trans in the late 1970s, while a significant number of respondents encountered issues within mental health services, such as having their gender identity treated as a symptom of mental distress, being asked inappropriate questions about their sexual behaviour and being told that their mental health issues were due to them being trans. Not surprisingly, just under half of respondents who answered this question stated that they had avoided urgent help or support when distressed because of being trans, and around a further quarter would have concerns about accessing support in the future. While there have been considerable changes in society regarding trans people, particularly around ensuring protections and an equitable service, previous negative experiences may still haunt respondents and make them weary of contacting mental health services for support. As such, earlier negative experiences can have an impact upon mental health later in life.

The majority of respondents had less than ideal informal sources of support on account of their trans status. Some respondents referred to the isolation and penalties they faced as a result of transitioning in terms of being forced to relocate (from jobs, houses, etc.), relationship break-ups and the need for a 'fresh start' elsewhere, resulted in the severing of community and financial ties. In addition, 43 per cent of those with children reported seeing their children less or losing contact with their children altogether as a result of being trans. This is especially worrying, not least because vital support in later life is significantly reduced.

However, elsewhere, comments suggest that, in the absence of biological families and relationship break-ups, trans friends and support networks may be coming into their own as crucial sources of social support for older trans people. This, combined with the positive relationship that respondents revealed to their own trans identity, suggests resilience and endurance in the face of haphazard formal sources of support and kinship structures.

Clearly much needs to be done to reassure older trans people that they can access mainstream mental health services without fear of being treated negatively or experiencing discrimination and prejudice. Support also needs to be in place to assist families in coming to terms with their loved one's gender identity. In addition, of the utmost importance is targeted work which supports older trans people in navigating the wider structures of health care, bolstering them to be equipped to deal with the combined processes of ageing and transition, ageism and transphobia, as well as to manage the nuances of transgenderism in later life.

Note

1 'Trans' is used here as an abbreviation and an umbrella term to refer to people whose gender identity differs from the one assigned to them at birth. It covers a range of gender identities – including those assigned 'female' at birth but who identify as men and those assigned 'male' at birth but who identify as women, as well as those who identify with both genders (bi-gender) and those who identify outside of the binary gender system of male/female (non-binary). It also includes those who cross-dress or who identify as transvestite.

References

Ansara, YG. (2015) 'Challenging cisgenderism in the ageing and aged care sector: Meeting the needs of older people of trans and/or non-binary experience', *Australasian Journal on Ageing,* 34(S2): 14–18.

Bailey, L. (2012) 'Trans ageing: Thoughts on a life course approach in order to better understand trans lives', in Ward, R, Rivers. I. and Sutherland, M. (eds), *Lesbian, Gay, Bisexual and Transgender Ageing: Biographical Approaches for Inclusive Care and Support.* London: Jessica Kingsley Publishers, pp. 51–66.

Fredriksen-Goldsen, KI., Cook-Daniels, L., Kim, H-J. et al. (2014) 'Physical and mental health of transgender older adults: An at-risk and underserved population', *The Gerontologist,* 54(3): 488–500.

Green, J. and Thorogood, N. (2004) *Qualitative Methods for Health Research.* London: Sage.

Hendricks, ML. and Testa, RJ. (2012) 'A conceptual framework for clinical work with transgender and gender nonconforming clients: An adaptation of the Minority Stress Model', *Professional Psychology: Research and Practice,* 43(5): 460–467.

McNeil, J., Bailey, L., Ellis, S. et al. (2012) *Trans Mental Health Study.* Sheffield: Sheffield Hallam University.

Riggs, DW., Ansara, GY. and Treharne, GJ. (2015) 'An evidence-based model for understanding the mental health experiences of transgender Australians', *Australian Psychologist,* 50(1): 32–39.

Rood, BA., Reisner, SL., Surace, FI. et al. (2016) 'Expecting rejection: Understanding the minority stress experiences of transgender and gender-nonconforming individuals', *Transgender Health,* 1(1): 151–164.

Warren, JC., Smalley, KB. and Barefoot, KN. (2016) 'Psychological well-being among transgender and genderqueer individuals', *International Journal of Transgenderism,* 17(3–4): 114–123.

Witten, TM. (2014) 'It's not all darkness: Robustness, resilience, and successful transgender aging', *LGBT Health,* 1(1): 24–33.

5 Trans temporalities and non-linear ageing

Ruth Pearce

[T]ransgender lives may require mixed strategies – not only healing and an achieved coherence but also the ability to represent and to inhabit temporal, gendered, and conceptual discontinuities.

Kadji Amin

At the time of writing, I am 10 years old, 14 years old, and 30 years old. I was born 30 years ago; in chronological terms, I have lived for 30 years. Chronological time is, however, just one means by which ageing may be understood (Baars, 1997). When we talk about age in terms of chronological time, we make a number of assumptions. Most importantly, we assume that our journey through the life course is linear, progressing from birth (at the beginning of the journey) to death (at the end). But my age may also be understood in terms of *trans time*. As a trans woman, I have experienced non-linear temporalities of disruption, disjuncture and discontinuity.

By temporality, I refer to 'the *social* patterning of experiences and understandings of time' (Amin, 2014: 219, emphasis added). Through conceptualising time as a social phenomenon, we might think about other beginnings and other ends, as well as wider temporal shifts and discontinuities across the life course. It is not unusual for trans people to do this: for example, through talking about age in terms of *trans years* in addition to years since birth. What if we were to regard my coming out at the age of 16 as a beginning (and, for that matter, as an end to my 'previous' life)? In this case, I might say that I am 14 years old in trans years. This does not, of course, change my chronological age: I am both 14 *and* 30. Or, we might regard my commencement of hormone therapy as a beginning, in which case I am 10 (but also still 14 and 30).

Importantly, trans years are not necessarily linked to chronological years. For instance, two different trans people who are both aged 80 in chronological years may have aged quite differently in trans years: perhaps one of them came out many decades ago, while the other has only been out for a couple of years. These individuals are likely to have had vastly different trans temporal experiences, which belie their apparently similar chronological age.

In this chapter I explore the consequences of trans temporalities for ageing. Non-linear ageing is not simply a matter of theory, but an approach which can enable us to 'do justice to the complex ways in which people inhabit gender variance' (Amin, 2014, p. 219). As Bailey and colleagues note (Chapter 4, this volume), trans people tend to face a range of specific challenges as they age, and may fear accessing mainstream forms of care, such as mental health services. It is therefore vital that academics and service providers alike understand how temporal phenomena such as trans years can shape trans identities and experiences.

I begin by outlining theories of queer and trans temporality that help make sense of community terminology such as 'trans years'. I then show how trans people may experience ageing in a variety of quite different ways, drawing upon a range of literature as well as findings from two qualitative research projects. Finally, I detail two common features of non-linear trans ageing: anticipation and delayed adolescence. These discussions draw primarily upon evidence, issues and challenges that have been identified in Western European and North American research.

Straight, queer and trans temporalities

What does a 'normal' life course look like? Experiences differ enormously from individual to individual. However, in the West we tend to assume that certain life events will (or otherwise *should*) take place at key points in a person's life, according to a linear narrative that progresses alongside chronological ageing. As a child, the 'normal' individual will be brought up by their (heterosexual) parents and educated within an institution. As an adolescent, they will explore new feelings and experiences, and learn to become independent. As a young adult, they will take a job. Maybe they will also fall in love (typically, with a single person of the 'opposite' sex), in which case they may be expected to marry their lover, settle down together in a shared home, and eventually have their own children in turn. In later life they will enjoy retirement, and may require specialist care in their final years.

Within this model, it is apparent that many things will change irreversibly as a person ages; the individual can anticipate these seemingly inevitable changes in their life through imagining a future that is bound to follow from their experience of the present. However, certain other aspects of the self – such as sexuality, gender and sexed embodiment – remain fixed. This linear, (re)productive temporality has been described as *straight time* (Muñoz, 2007). While a great many individuals' lives deviate from the constraints of straight time, this model provides a normative narrative by which we might frame our expectations and assumptions about the life course.

Queer time helps make sense of what may happen when a person's life can no longer be understood through these 'temporal frames of bourgeois reproduction and family, longevity [...] and inheritance' (Halberstam, 2005, p.6). Queer time is an asynchronous temporality, in which ageing and experience do not necessarily proceed according to normative expectations. For instance, Halberstam (2005, p. 153) describes how childless queers may experience a 'stretched-out adolescence' through long-term involvement in subcultural activities such as punk music and fashion, thereby challenging 'the conventional binary formulation of a life narrative divided by a clear break between youth and adulthood'.[1]

Trans individuals often experience asynchronous disruptions of the life course, leading them to inhabit queer temporalities. Halberstam (2005) explores the example of Brandon Teena, who departed from normative anticipations of heterosexual ageing associated with being raised as a girl in a small, rural American settlement, by moving to another town and starting a new life as a man. In constructing this new life for himself, Teena also created a new history in which he had been born and raised as male. However, his assigned gender was later discovered by acquaintances, leading to his murder at the age of 21. Teenas's life departed from the linear norms of straight time in numerous ways, with new beginnings, a reimagined past, and his life cut tragically short before any opportunity to age as an adult. While he died young, many trans people continue to experience queer temporal discontinuities into later life.

Fabbre (2015) notes that discourses around 'successful' ageing tend to assume not only that older people are heterosexual and cis,[2] but also that they have lived heterosexual lives in accordance with the gender they were assigned at birth. These are *cisgenderist* discourses (Ansara, 2015). Like heterosexism, cisgenderism describes how even unintentional and well-intentioned assumptions and practices can work to shut down certain possibilities with regard to gendered and sexual expression on a *systemic and structural* level; this contrasts with transphobia, 'which emphasises individual hostility and negative attitudes' (Ansara, 2015, p. 15). If a chronologically older individual underwent significant social and/or physical changes at an earlier age, through *transitioning* to their preferred or felt gender from that which they were assigned at birth, their experiences stand in contrast to the cisgenderist norms of straight time. Others may challenge normative expectations of ageing by experimenting with their gender, changing their appearance and/or transitioning in later life.

Halberstam's (2005) conceptualisation of queer time tends to emphasise the present rather than the future, looking to the moment rather than anticipating what might yet come to be. However, other accounts of trans temporality emphasise anticipation, futurity and/or the continual interplay of past/present/future. In her empirical study of trans video blogs, Horak (2014) describes how individuals undergoing a physical transition construct alternative narratives of temporal progress, which she describes as 'hormone time'. Hormone time 'begins with the first shot of testosterone or HRT pills (hormone replacement therapy) and is measured against that date, even years afterward' (Horak, 2014, p. 579). In this sense, it describes a similar phenomenon to that of trans years, in which trans people employ an alternative chronology to make sense of their lives. By contrast, Carter (2013) highlights the potential non-linearity of social and bodily change through his account of 'transitional time', which describes how the trans body may carry traces of a differently gendered past and/or anticipate a differently gendered future. In inhabiting transitioning or transitioned bodies, trans people may be understood to engage in 'dynamic and relational negotiations of wrongness', in which '[a]nticipation, retroflexion, and continuity co-exist in the same body, at the same moving moment of space and time' (Carter, 2013, p. 141).

These differing accounts of trans temporality do not stand in opposition to one another. Rather, they provide insights into the various ways in which trans people might experience time: experiences that often contrast with chronological and straight notions of linear progression.

Methods

I turn next to look at how these theories may be employed to better understand the specific experiences of chronologically older trans people, grounding my discussion in three sources of empirical data. First, I provide a critical review of existing literature on trans ageing and the lives of older trans people. Secondly and thirdly, I draw upon data from two of my own qualitative research projects: 'Genderforking' (Pearce, 2012) and 'Understanding Trans Health' (Pearce, 2018). From these sources, I have identified several arenas in which theories of trans temporality can help us understand the experiences and challenges faced by chronologically older trans people, as well as a range of indicative empirical examples which I outline to illustrate how particular phenomena can play out in practice.

For the 'Genderforking' project, I undertook a retrospective analysis of posts and discussion threads on the international (but primarily Western/ Anglophone) community blog Genderfork[3] from 2007 to 2010. My focus was on how gender ambiguity and diversity were explored and expressed by Genderfork contributors. 'Understanding Trans Health' was an online ethnographic project, entailing participant observation of UK-based trans community forums, trans activist groups and health professional websites and literatures between 2010 and 2017. My analysis focused on how discourses of trans health are understood differently and negotiated within and between these spaces. I employed a thematic approach to data analysis for both projects (Braun and Clarke, 2006). While neither project originally focused specifically on older trans people or trans ageing, I identified a number of themes relating to trans temporalities, which inform my discussion in this chapter.

Ageing in different times

Chronologically older trans people form an extremely diverse population. In addition to differences in identity and life experience arising from factors such as gender identity, class, dis/ability, ethnicity and race, nationality, and religion, older trans people have also variously come to terms with *being* trans at different ages (Bailey, 2012; Porter et al., 2016). Individual trans elders may or may not have come out and/or transitioned (or, indeed, de-transitioned or re-transitioned) at some point in their lives, and those who have done so will have done this at quite different ages. Consequently, they are likely to have had very different experiences of *being* trans, depending on *when* they came out and/or transitioned. Siverskog (2014, p. 391) therefore argues that in order to understand the experiences of older trans people, 'it is crucial to understand their previous experiences of (trans)gender identities during life, and how these are intertwined with the historical context'.

The literature on trans ageing often discusses the experiences of chronologically older trans people in terms of those who came out earlier in their lives, and those who have come out more recently (Bailey, 2012; Cook-Daniels, 2006). This model encourages us to acknowledge how older trans people who came out while they were young (i.e. those who are older in trans years as well as in chronological years) are likely to have had very different experiences to those who are younger in trans years. For example, Siverskog describes the challenges faced by interviewee Klas:

> Klas, who transitioned in the '70s, experienced a transition that was different to how it would be today. To get the diagnosis, he had to go to a gynecologist, which can be very difficult for someone not comfortable with their [assigned] sex. He also had to be institutionalized in a mental hospital for one week, during which time he underwent many psychological tests.
>
> (Siverskog 2014, p. 297)

In other countries, such as the United States, many individuals seeking to transition were historically required to cut contact with their family and friends and – in a similar manner to Brandon Teena – effectively start a completely new life as a 'stealth' transsexual (Meyerowitz, 2002).

While transitioning individuals continue to face significant challenges in accessing health care services, the especially draconian measures described by Siverskog and Meyerowitz are no longer routinely imposed upon trans people in most North American and Western European contexts.[4] These are, however, experiences that have had significant long-term impacts upon the mental health and forms of support available to the people who have undergone them.

In addition to facing more traumatic experiences upon coming out or embarking upon transition, chronologically older trans people are likely to have experienced significant challenges across their life course. On average, they will have encountered more instances of discrimination and victimisation than cis LGB people of the same age, and are also more likely to experience poorer physical health and/or be disabled (Fredriksen-Goldsen et al., 2013).

In addition, like cis LGB people, some older trans people will have survived the AIDS crisis, and will have undergone the ordeal of countless members of their community dying of mysterious causes at a time of heightened prejudice. For trans people experiencing intersecting forms of marginalisation – such as disabled trans people, or trans people of colour – such traumatic experiences are likely to be more common and more severe (Chang and Singh, 2016; Porter et al., 2016).

Trans lives are not, of course, defined only by difficulty and trauma. Trans people who have had the opportunity to live for many years or decades in their preferred gender(s) will have experienced numerous advantages as well as challenges. Horak (2014, p. 579) describes how trans people moving into hormone time depict 'a heroic journey of coming into oneself, moving from fear, deception, and self-hatred to joy, authenticity, and confidence'. While the initial rush of excitement that can come with transition may fade with time, the long-term advantages do not. McNeil and colleagues (2012, p. 16) note that transition can have an enormous impact upon trans people's life satisfaction, with 70 per cent of survey respondents indicating that they were more satisfied with their lives since transitioning; in comparison, 2 per cent stated that they were less satisfied. Transition is also related to improved body satisfaction, less avoidance of public and social spaces, a decrease in mental health service use, and reduced suicide and self-harm (McNeil et al., 2012, p. 83). In Chapter 4 (this volume), Bailey and colleagues further observe that chronologically older trans people have reported better rates of mental health when compared to the wider trans population.

Siverskog (2014, p. 391) therefore argues that for individuals such as Klas, who transitioned earlier in life, the context of coming out and transitioning 'differs from the context in which younger transgender people are now growing up'. However, this context is also one in which trans people who are older in chronological years but *younger* in trans years are also coming to terms with being trans. Such individuals are therefore likely to share certain experiences with trans people who are chronologically younger. In addition to navigating similar legal and social systems upon coming out, beginning transition and/or entering hormone time, they are likely to have a knowledge and awareness of trans politics similarly grounded in the events and concerns of the present and recent past.

In some instances, chronologically younger trans individuals may be considerably *older* in trans years than chronologically older trans people. In such cases, chronologically older trans individuals may seek the knowledge and experience of those 'younger' individuals who came out and/or transitioned before them. Examples of this may be seen on Genderfork, where on one occasion a contributor asked:

> Young people: what advice would you give your closeted gender-variant elders yearning to be free after years of forced passing?
>
> (Tab)[5]

This query elicited a range of responses from the blog's readers. Some chronologically younger contributors, such as Lilybean, encouraged chronologically older readers to embrace their felt identity. In turn, a number of middle-aged and older contributors, such as Renae Ann, expressed their gratitude for this advice:

> It's NEVER too late. It's NEVER useless. The strength is there and always will be there, the issue is tapping it [...] being yourself is the best you can do for the world.
>
> (Lilybean)

> I'm 55, and I've only recently begun to be able to explore my situation in even a small way. I just now discovered this forum and really appreciate that a question like this can even get asked. Thank you so very much. [...] Your advice is good, and I can sense behind it a gentle thoughtfulness. '[...] it's never too late to make a change' [...]yes, absolutely – that is ever so true.
>
> (Renae Ann)

In this way, queer discontinuities within a trans life course may disrupt normative assumptions about the relative accumulation of knowledge and experience among chronologically older and younger individuals.

However, people coming out later in life will also have unique experiences that arise at the intersection of their chronological age and trans trajectory. Using Carter's (2013) description of transitional time, we can understand these individuals' experiences as being shaped by the temporal intersections of continuity and change, the social and the physical, trans youth and chronological age. For example, Siverskog (2014) describes how her research participants saw both advantages and disadvantages in coming out in later life. Coming out in retirement can circumvent concerns about negative reactions from bosses and colleagues, but can also result in isolation, particularly if the individual is rejected by family members. Physical elements of chronological age may have an impact upon gender performance:

> Some felt that the body became more androgynous with age and others perceived bodily aging to be problematic for their possibilities of performing gender. Wrinkles, the inability to walk in high heels, and different shapes of the body were all mentioned as potential complications for gender performance.
>
> (Siverskog, 2014, p. 393)

Chronologically older trans people seeking affirmation in their preferred gender may also encounter prejudice at the intersection of transphobia, cisgenderism and ageism, from carers, family members and medical practitioners who feel that they are 'too old' to transition or to express their gender differently (Siverskog, 2014; Ansara, 2015).

Consequently, it is important to acknowledge that certain forms of knowledge and experience are highly specific to chronologically older trans people. Creating links and building community among individuals with these specific experiences can be particularly beneficial, as Genderfork user nick notes:

> So I'd say that the best thing an older genderqueer could do is get in touch with other older genderqueer[s] and look for their experience. They're likely to go through the same things, same dilemmas. [...] it's never too late to make a change. Even if you're 90, the years you can still live in your life are precious and best spent being yourself.
>
> (nick)

Of course, trans people do not necessarily come out or transition *either* in their chronological youth *or* in later life. Any given trans person may have come out at any point during their life course. Moreover, the time at which a person comes out or transitions does not necessarily align with the time at which they become 'visibly' trans. While some trans people move through the world *as* trans after coming out, others may effectively 'disappear' for decades through going stealth and passing as cis, only to 'reappear' in order to access trans-specific services or due to increased vulnerability (for instance, being outed by care workers) at a later chronological age (Cook-Daniels, 2006; Witten, 2017).

The differing experiences of trans elders may therefore be understood as the outcome of myriad queerly intersecting temporalities and socio-historical contexts, reflecting rapidly changing social, political and legal circumstances for trans people. The past century has seen enormous shifts in these arenas, which have only accelerated in the past three decades following the emergence of the trans liberation movement in the early 1990s.

Anticipation: living in limbo

A key element of trans community discourse identified during the 'Understanding Trans Health' project was that of *anticipation*: orientation towards an uncertain future, mediated through trans people's experience of the present as a liminal or transitional space (Pearce, 2018). In the UK, transitioning patients' discourses of anticipation are typically shaped by long waiting lists for gender identity services, as well as worries and hopes about what might happen when these services are finally accessed. Community discussions around the availability of health care and the challenges that patients may face – including transphobia and cisgenderism from service providers – can lead to individuals feeling disempowered and fearful before they even have an opportunity to attend an appointment with a gender identity specialist.

In the meantime they may feel trapped in a form of limbo, having recognised that they experience dysphoric feelings but being unable to take steps towards addressing this, at least not through formal medical services. I argue that in the context of anticipation, the temporal disruptions of queer and transitional time are not necessarily welcome, even as trans patients may look forward to the desired relief of physical transition.

People who come out or transition while chronologically older are likely to have lived in a time of anticipation for many decades. Ansara (2015) and Siverskog (2014) describe how research participants remained closeted for a very long time because they were scared about the potential consequences of having their gender identity discovered by colleagues, partners, family members or friends. In this way, cisgenderist norms can effectively act as 'a prison' (Siverskog 2014, p. 392), with the anticipation of a fearful future outweighing hope, keeping trans people trapped within the limbo of the closet, unable to fully express themselves. Negative responses from family members who discover a trans person's identity can also play a role in preventing or substantially delaying that person's transition (Cook-Daniels, 2006; Ansara, 2015). This can lead to trans people internalising anti-trans stigma and feelings of shame, causing past incidents of being outed or abused to resonate through the years. Some individuals may further feel that even if they were to transition, they cannot be who they really want to be. For instance, 'Understanding Trans Health' participant Ellie describes how her worries about how she might be perceived by herself and others following transition led her to delay embodied change for decades:

> I had serious doubts about the transsexual path in my youth. I buried, denied and ran away from it for 40 years because I wanted to be A WOMAN – not 'a transsexual'. But here I am, at 58 years old and 2 years post-op. I finally feel peace in my soul, but it's really late and my life is almost over.
>
> (Ellie)[6]

Ellie's experiences reflect those of several of Siverskog's (2014) research participants, who similarly described a historic discomfort with the medical language of transsexualism, and a sense of loss from living in limbo for so long.

In many cases, therefore, trans people feel that they *cannot* anticipate a desirable post-closet future, yet their lives remain constrained by this future that may never come. Nevertheless, this is not necessarily an experience that has to last forever. Trans people who do come out and begin to live their life in a manner that affirms their gender identity may be understood to have moved beyond the unwanted queer disruptions that come with time of anticipation. Indeed, Horak (2014) describes hormone time as a temporality that offers an alternative, liberated form of linearity, one that is importantly different but comparable to straight time.

However, trans people who transitioned long ago may effectively re-enter a time of anticipation as they begin to contemplate losing some of their independence towards the end of their lives. As Witten (2014) notes, trans people requiring specialised care arrangements in the latter stages of their lives can face numerous challenges due to transphobia and cisgenderism within a range of settings, both within the home and in institutions such as private care homes or hospitals. Stigmatising anti-trans behaviour such as discrimination and misgendering are endemic within health care systems (Pearce, 2018); this is no less the case within elderly care settings, where scholars of trans gerontology have described how trans people may face degendering, harassment and sexual violence from carers and/or family members (Cook-Daniels, 2006; Ansara, 2015; Witten, 2017). Chronologically older trans people are therefore likely to express significant concerns around their ability to function independently in later life. In the US TransMetLife Survey, participants were invited to rank order a list of concerns about ageing: the top four concerns listed were all related to this issue of independence, with participants particularly concerned about 'becoming unable to care for myself; becoming sick or disabled; becoming dependent upon others; and becoming confused or demented' (Witten, 2017, p. 34).

With their projected future shaped by a significant and not undergrounded fear of vulnerability, some chronologically older trans people plan drastic actions. One option for trans people in this situation is to 're-closet', or hide their gender identity; another is to 'de-transition', or shift back towards living in the gender they were assigned at birth (Siverskog, 2014; Porter et al., 2016). Both approaches are likely to prove traumatic and may cut the individual off from trans community support, but can also protect them from specific forms of anticipated transphobic violence. In other instances, chronologically older trans people plan 'self-euthanasia' or suicide to avoid entering long-term care (Witten, 2014).

The time of anticipation is therefore defined by perceptions of an uncertain future, even as trans people experiencing this temporality prior to transition may remain caught in a continuous present, a form of limbo. Entering the comparative certainty of hormone time can offer a sense of linearity, affirmation and peace, as much in (chronological) middle or older age as in (chronological) youth. However, in later life individuals who have transitioned may find themselves facing an uncertain and fearful future.

Atemporal adolescence

Halberstam's (2005, p. 153) description of the 'stretched-out adolescence' of queer time draws primarily upon queer people's engagements in activities and interests that are normatively associated with adolescence, such as hip-hop, punk rock, fashion, and promiscuous or polyamorous sexual activity. Halberstam associates queer people's engagement in these activities with a rejection of normative modes of life progression and reproductive responsibilities (such as for children or grandchildren) that accumulate within straight time.

Trans people who seek to transition socially and/or medically frequently experience a different kind of queer 'adolescence'. This experience coincides with the first months or years of transition, and typically involves the kinds of social experimentation and physical changes that are associated with teenage years in the context of straight time. Bailey (2012) and Ansara (2015) describe this as a 'second puberty', noting that trans people may learn (or unlearn) certain 'gender-appropriate' social behaviours, find new social networks and experiment with new clothing. During this time, trans men and other transmasculine individuals in particular may look younger than they actually are: as Schilt (2006, p. 484) notes, 'without facial hair or visible stubble, [these individuals] are often taken to be young boys, a mistake that intensifies with the onset of hormone therapy and the development of peach fuzz that marks the beginning of facial hair growth'. This is an atemporal rather than 'stretched out' adolescence: it sits outside of the normative linear narrative of straight time, which assumes that a single puberty takes place during the teen years before an individual progresses into adulthood.

Consequently, trans individuals who come out or transition later in life may have specific desires, or experiences of uncertainty and experimentation, more typically associated with adolescence. For this reason, Ansara (2015) asserts that chronological age is not always the most useful conceptual approach for understanding trans people's needs. He illustrates this with an example from an interview with Maggie, a residential aged care provider who supported Nancy, a trans woman, in expressing herself following initial mistreatment from other care workers.

> Nancy dressed very inappropriately when I first met her. The staff used to think it was funny when she walked out in a bikini with half her genitals falling out the bottom of her bikini pants. They thought it was funny to watch her get around like that. When I took over the place I fired the lot of them and helped Nancy to feminise herself. We were teaching her how to be feminine and she blossomed.
>
> ('Maggie', quoted in Ansara, 2015, p. 17)

Ansara argues that while women such as Nancy are often pathologised, with their gendered feelings and attempts at self-expression attributed to cognitive decline, they can in fact benefit from being afforded the opportunity and support to express themselves in line with their gendered desires.

Like the teenage adolescence of straight time, the second puberty that many trans people experience may be a passing phase of life experience or personal development, associated with the early years of hormone time (Schilt, 2006; Horak, 2014). However, it can also have more of a long-term impact upon trans people's experiences of age and ageing. While Schilt (2006, p. 484) argues that transmasculine individuals ultimately tend to 'age into' their differently gendered appearance, in my research I noted that trans people of all genders often maintain a somewhat 'youthful' appearance that contrasts with their chronological age, reflecting Carter's (2013) observations regarding the embodied co-existence of youth/age and past/present/future within transitional time. For some – particularly transmasculine individuals who choose not to undergo hormone therapy – this can be an effect of transitioning socially without undertaking particular medical procedures. For others, however, medical interventions such as facial feminisation surgery or high hormone levels during the early years of second adolescence can effectively have a long-term rejuvenating effect. The effects of this can sometimes be surprising even to trans people themselves, as may be seen in the following examples from a conversation that took place on a community forum I visited for the 'Understanding Trans Health' project. In this instance, Alain – a 63-year-old trans man – shared a YouTube video of himself talking about his experiences. Following an initial conversation about the video, the topic of Alain's age came up, leading other forum users to express surprise at his relatively youthful appearance in both the video and the avatar (profile picture) he used on the forum.

> Alain, you didn't have an age on your forum profile and the pic makes you look years younger so I was coming at this [conversation] from a misconceived perception.
>
> (Ben)

> Based on your video, I'd have said you were late-40s, early 50s. But not 63 though man, congratulations, lol!
>
> (Aiden)

The atemporal adolescence of second puberty can therefore play an important role in shaping trans people's relationship with time and ageing, both in terms of social experience and its mediation through physical appearance. This can have a range of impacts upon how chronologically older trans people might appear to others, as well as upon their desires and needs.

Conclusion

In a poetic description of transitional temporalities, Carter (2013, p. 141) declares that 'transition wraps the body in the folds of social time'. In this chapter, I have shown how queer and trans temporalities can significantly shape experiences of age and ageing, in ways that frequently depart from normative, linear and 'straight' understandings of time. Through actions such as coming out and transitioning (or potentially re-transitioning/detransitioning), trans people encounter embodied social forms of temporal disjuncture, beginning their lives anew in one sense (or multiple senses) while experiencing continuity (through chronological ageing) in another. Trans experiences of time can be characterised by features such as new and atemporal experiences of the present, as may be seen in a second puberty with the onset of transition; or a focus on an imagined future, such as through powerfully anticipating anti-trans discrimination, access to trans-specific care and/or the challenges of long-term care in later life. Such discontinuities can happen at any time in the life course, meaning that different trans people in later life will often have had dramatically different experiences of ageing and being trans, depending on when they came out and how the consequences of this were experienced.

Thinking through the complexities of trans temporalities can therefore help us understand how trans lives and trans ageing might differ substantially from cis lives and cis ageing in particular ways; moreover, it can also illustrate how trans lives and ageing vary greatly among different trans people. This way of thinking is important because it can help us capture the nuances of trans ageing and better understand the sometimes extreme challenges that trans people face as they age.

Notes

1 This is not to say that all LGBT or queer people live within queer time. In the wake of important social and political changes regarding marriage, adoption and in vitro fertilisation, straight time may also increasingly be understood as the basis of a homonormative life course model.
2 The term 'cis' describes individuals whose gender identity and gender expression broadly align with the gender they were assigned at birth. This usually contrasts with the experience of trans people.
3 http://genderfork.com.
4 In some other contexts (e.g. Eastern European countries such as Ukraine) individuals hoping to transition are still institutionalised in mental hospitals for assessment as a matter of course.
5 Genderfork is a public blog, and users are aware that their contributions and comments can be seen by anyone. For material from the 'Genderforking' project, I have therefore reproduced the pseudonyms chosen by the individual users.
6 The quotes used in this chapter from the 'Understanding Trans Health' project originated from private, member-only spaces. I obtained informed consent from participants to reproduce their comments, and also use pseudonyms.

References

Amin, K. (2014) 'Temporality', *TSQ: Transgender Studies Quarterly*, 1(1–2): 219–222.
Ansara, YG. (2015) 'Challenging cisgenderism in the ageing and aged care sector: Meeting the needs of older people of trans and/or non-binary experience', *Australasian Journal on Ageing*, 34(S2): 14–18.
Baars, J. (1997) 'Concepts of time and narrative temporality in the study of aging', *Journal of Aging Studies*, 11(4): 283–295.
Bailey, L. (2012) 'Trans life course and ageing – some thoughts on a life course approach in order to better understand trans lives', in Ward, R., Rivers, I. and Sutherland, M. (eds), *Lesbian, Gay, Bisexual and Transgender Ageing: Biographical Approaches for Inclusive Support*. London: Jessica Kingsley, pp. 51–66.

Braun, V. and Clarke, V. (2006) 'Using thematic analysis in psychology', *Qualitative Research in Psychology*, 3(2): 77–101.

Carter, J. (2013) 'Embracing transition, or dancing in the folds of time', in Stryker, S. and Aizura, AZ. (eds), *The Transgender Studies Reader 2*. New York: Routledge, pp. 130–143.

Chang, SC. and Singh, AA. (2016) 'Affirming psychological practice with transgender and gender nonconforming people', *Psychology of Sexual Orientation and Gender Diversity*, 3(2): 140–147.

Cook-Daniels, L. (2006) 'Trans aging', in Kimmel, D., Rose, T. and David, S. (eds), *Lesbian, Gay, Bisexual, and Transgender Aging: Research and Clinical Perspectives*. New York: Columbia University Press, pp. 20–35.

Fabbre, VD. (2015) 'Gender transitions in later life: A queer perspective on successful aging', *The Gerontologist*, 55(1): 144–153.

Fredriksen-Goldsen, KI., Cook-Daniels, L., Kim, H-J., Erosheva, EA., Emlet, CA., Hoy-Ellis, CP., Goldsen, J. and Muraco, A. (2014) 'Physical and mental health of transgender older adults: An at-risk and underserved population', *The Gerontologist*, 54(3): 488–500.

Halberstam, J. (2005) *In a Queer Time and Place: Transgender Bodies, Subcultural Lives*. New York: New York University Press.

Horak, L. (2014) 'Trans on Youtube: Intimacy, visibility, temporality', *TSQ: Transgender Studies Quarterly*, 1(4): 472–585.

McNeil, J., Bailey, L., Ellis, S., Morton, J. and Regan, M. (2012) *Trans Mental Health Study 2012*. Edinburgh: Equality Network.

Meyerowitz, J. (2002) *How Sex Changed: A History of Transsexuality in the United States*. Cambridge, MA: Harvard University Press.

Muñoz, JE. (2007) 'Cruising the toilet: LeRoi Jones/Amiri Baraka, radical Black traditions, and queer futurity', *GLQ: A Journal of Lesbian and Gay Studies*, 13(2): 353–367.

Pearce, R. (2012) 'Inadvertent praxis: What can "Genderfork" tell us about trans feminism?', *MP: An Online Feminist Journal*, 3(4): 87–129.

Pearce, R. (2018) *Understanding Trans Health: Discourse, Power and Possibility*. Bristol: Policy Press.

Porter, KE., Brennan-Ing, M., Chang, SC., dickey, lm., Singh, AA., Bower, KL. and Witten, TM. (2016) 'Providing competent and affirming services for transgender and gender nonconforming older adults', *Clinical Gerontologist*, 39(5): 366–388.

Schilt, K. (2006) 'Just one of the guys? How transmen make gender visible at work', *Gender and Society*, 20(4): 465–490.

Siverskog, A. (2014) '"They just don't have a clue": Transgender aging and implications for social work', *Journal of Gerontological Social Work*, 57(2–4): 386–406.

Witten, TM. (2014) 'End of life, chronic illness, and trans-identities', *Journal of Social Work in End-of-Life & Palliative Care*, 10(1): 34–58.

Witten, TM. (2017) 'Health and well-being of transgender elders', *Annual Review of Gerontology and Geriatrics*, 37(1): 27–41.

6 Levels and layers of invisibility

Exploring the intersections of
ethnicity, culture and religion in
the lives of older LGBT people

Joanne McCarthy and Roshan das Nair

Introduction

The proliferation of research literature around the diversity within lesbian, gay, bisexual and trans (LGBT) communities often focuses on *one* identity characteristic (e.g. ethnicity and sexuality), but not on more than one. Therefore, the issues of LGBT people who are identify as 'older' *and* as 'ethnic minority' are less well understood. Being older, non-heterosexual and an ethnic minority form specific sites of invisibility and we know little about the impact of this invisibility in terms of significant life markers/events (e.g. relationships, parenting, bereavement), and access to support and care. This is an area that is becoming increasingly important and urgent to investigate given that there are rising numbers of older LGBT people in an overall ageing population, and this will increasingly include ethnic minorities.

In this chapter, we aim to explore research in this area that covers three concepts (ethnicity, religion and culture) and how these intersect alongside people's sexual expressions, desires and/or identities and being older.

The chapter offers insights into the experiences such groups would have had (and have). Older LGBT people may not find it easy to disclose such experiences, but nonetheless these may continue to affect them; and their current concerns and ways of coping. We conclude by reflecting on some of the challenges researchers face in connecting with those who are less seen and less heard than others in society, and possible ways to overcome these challenges.

At the outset, we would like to present a conundrum. What terms do we use to describe people's sexual expressions, desires and/or identities, and by the same token, what terms do we use to describe their ethnicity or ethnic grouping? These are important questions because we are seeking to understand the lives of ethnic groups and older generations who may not associate with LGBT identities (especially if growing up in a culture and time when these identities were stigmatised and vilified). In this chapter, we have chosen not to use the terms Black and Minority Ethnic (BME) or Black, Asian and Minority Ethnic (BAME), because although these terms are used in surveys or for other data-collection purposes, the specific labelling of several groups of people as 'Black' or 'Asian' is problematic. Indeed, various people (including Trevor Phillips, the former chairperson of the UK Commission for Racial Equality) have called for the abandonment of the BME and BAME terms (The Guardian, 2015). Some suggest alternatives, such as 'people of colour' or 'visible minorities', but these too obfuscate the experiences of those who do not identify, or are not identified (by others), as being Black or Asian. Therefore, we use the term 'ethnic minority'.[1] We have chosen to use the term LGBT (and associated identities), because much of the research uses this term consistently, but where 'indigenous identities' or identity labels are used (or, indeed, where no identity labels are used), we present these as used by the researchers or participants (e.g. in places these may include LGB or LGBTQ), or use the term 'sexual minority' or 'non-heterosexual'.

Older, ethnic minority LGBT people: the research literature

To fully understand the lived experience of ethnic minority LGBT people, we need to view them in their gendered, sociocultural, historical and geographical context, and how these aspects interact with contemporary society. In this section, we consider how the research literature in this area captures these contexts and advances our knowledge of this population.

A 25-year review of ageing and sexual orientation (Fredriksen-Goldsen and Muraco, 2010) reviewed 58 papers that reported on primary research published in peer-reviewed journals between the years 1984 and 2008. Their operational definition of 'older' was anyone aged over 50 years. Only two of their included studies addressed transgender issues, "although findings specific to gender identity were not reported in the articles and thus are not included" (p. 396). Seventeen per cent of their included studies only had White participants, 59 per cent had mixed samples, and interestingly, 24 per cent of the included studies did not report the race or ethnicity of their participants. The findings from the review report positive and negative aspects of LGBT ageing, with some differences between genders. They also suggest factors that help or hinder what they term 'successful ageing'.

It is noteworthy that the review had only one paper which considered both ethnicity and sexuality within the context of ageing. David and Knight's (2008) study included 383 gay men aged 18 to 55 and older (35 per cent in the latter category), and they report that almost half of their sample was Black. They found that African American older gay men experienced significantly higher levels of ageism than did their White counterparts, higher levels of racism than did younger African American men, and higher levels of heteronormativity than did both White and younger African American men (David and Knight, 2008; Fredriksen-Goldsen and Muraco, 2010, p. 398).

Fredriksen-Goldsen and Muraco's (2010) review is useful in identifying different 'waves' of research foci over the 25-year period they investigated. The focus has shifted from dispelling the myth that older LGB people experience maladjusted ageing, to focusing on the psychosocial correlates of adjustment and functioning, to the social and community-based needs and experiences of older LGB people. These were essential first steps in gathering a critical mass of research-based findings around LGB older people in general. Fredriksen-Goldsen and Muraco (2010) identify the need for future research to examine the nuance of how older LGBT people's multiple identities interact and intersect to give them a unique place in society, which poses challenges and threats, but also opportunities and needs.

Using the same search terms as Fredriksen-Goldsen and Muraco's (2010) review, we searched Medline, PsycINFO and Embase from 2008 to 2016 (last search 8 February 2016), and found 815 articles (after removing duplicates). While it is beyond the scope of this chapter to present a thorough report of this review, we make a few notable points.

There were several papers that related to HIV, anti-retroviral medication and ageing. There are a few more studies on transgender ageing (e.g. Persson, 2009; Witten, 2015) compared to Fredriksen-Goldsen and Muraco's 2010 review. Studies examining older LGBT sexualities in different countries have also begun to emerge (e.g. McCann et al. (2013) in Ireland; Hayman (2011) in Canada; Horner et al. (2012) in Australia; Fokkema and Kuyper (2009) in The Netherlands). However, these studies do not necessarily deal with the issues that ethnic minorities face *within* each of these countries, and they do not necessarily focus on religion and culture.

Based on the title and citation scan of our returned articles, we were only able to discern three studies that explicitly researched the experiences of older LGBT ethnic minorities. We acknowledge that we did not carry out an exhaustive search of the literature, but it provides a brief overview of the state of affairs in researching older LGBT ethnic minority issues.

Haile and colleagues' (2011) paper analyses the narratives of 10 gay and bisexual 'Black' men living in poverty, over the age of 50 and living with HIV/AIDS in New York City. The study focused mainly on experiences of stigma. This included the ways in which stigma devalued and dehumanised the participants, treating them as "just one more body within institutions charged with their care" (p. 4), and how their poverty, 'non-normative sexuality' and Black ethnicity contributed to this experience – not just in health care settings but also in the Black Church, in colleges and on the streets.

Woody's (2014) phenomenological study explored the perceived social discrimination and alienation experienced by 15 older African American lesbians (N=11) and gay men (N=4) aged from 58 to 72 years. Woody identified participants feeling a 'sense of alienation in the African American community', with experiences of being an outcast within their own families and extended communities, and at home, work or college. Not surprisingly, many chose to conceal their sexual identity – some deciding to communicate this on a need-to-know basis. Even with disclosure, many disliked the terms lesbian or gay, preferring terms like 'woman who loves woman', or 'same-gender-loving' (p. 154). Woody's participants also reported experiences of discrimination and alienation from organised religion. Nevertheless, many of her participants were able to negotiate a way of connecting with God that did not cause a dissonance between their religion/spirituality and their sexuality. This resonates with findings from our study detailed below. While some of these themes have been endorsed by other studies of ethnic minority LGBT people of all age groups, Woody's participants also spoke about 'feelings of grief and loss related to aging', (p. 155). Again, this feeling was related to a sense of alienation and feeling insignificant in a 'throw-away society' (p. 156), and their older age was seen as attracting yet another 'ism' (ageism). There is a sense of becoming *invisible* in some of the narratives, and a feeling of being isolated from their own ethnic communities *but* also the wider LGBT society, and isolation caused because of their age (e.g. inability to drive). Similar themes are echoed in Woody's (2015) paper, based on interviews with 15 African American lesbians aged 57 to 72 years. These papers highlight the themes of minority stress and resilience, which bring a new dimension to the literature.

Religion and identity conflict: the research literature

Many studies have explored how religious spaces tend to be exclusive and can have a negative outlook on same-sex sexuality or bisexuality (Barnes and Meyer, 2012; Brennan-Ing et al., 2013). As outlined by Westwood (2016, p. 2), religious institutions are 'frequently sites of heteronormativity (the assumption that heterosexuality is the norm), heterosexism (the privileging of heterosexuality) and homophobia (prejudice and discrimination towards persons who are LGB)'. Consequently, this can create identity conflict for many religious LGBT individuals (Levy and Reeves, 2011; Beagan and Hattie, 2014). Conflicts vary widely, as different religions (or communities of worship) have contrasting views and stances on sexuality. Some religions may be said to take little interest in the private sexual lives of their followers, but it is nevertheless a broad truth that most mainstream world religions still hold to a public position formally opposed to homosexuality.

Beagan and Hattie (2014) found that research is scarce concerning LGBTQ people in faith traditions other than Christianity; however, their search of the literature uncovered that Judaism, Native spirituality, Buddhism and Hinduism are more welcoming than others (Porter et al., 2013; Schnoor, 2006; Westerfield, 2012). Hinduism and Buddhism tend to view 'homosexuality' primarily from the standpoint of its karmic effects. Jaspal (2012) found that Sikh and Hindu religions do not explicitly forbid homosexuality but their cultural norms do. The little research evidence available indicates that Muslim LGBTQ people experience considerable identity conflict stemming from both religious and cultural condemnation. In Jaspal's study of gay Indian men in Britain, Sikh and Hindu participants appeared less concerned about sin than their Muslim participants, and more concerned about loss of family and community. Many worried about disappointing or being rejected by families for failing to fulfil social expectations to establish a 'normal' family and procreate. In a study by Valentine and Waite (2012, p. 478), heterosexual Christians, Jews, Muslims and Hindus said that homosexuality was 'unnatural', they spoke of it "as transgressing a religious duty to procreate, and as a threat to the fabric of society because of its assumed connection with promiscuity and the dismantling of marriage".

Again, existing research on religion and LGBT populations has often been from the perspective of one identity characteristic (sexuality), therefore neglecting the 'older' identity. For some individuals the unquestioned dominance of religion in their communities has meant that older LGBT individuals grew up in a social context where a non-heterosexual identity was deemed unacceptable, abnormal and sinful. This has led to a legacy of silence and invisibility about the religious lives of older LGBT individuals.

Older LGBT individuals have experienced considerable social and cultural shifts in their lifetimes. Much progress has been made over the past few decades in recognising and supporting LGBT people in many countries in contrast to times when being gay was imbued with stigma and shame (Barrett, 2008).

Discovering that one is attracted to someone of the same sex in an environment characterised by anti-LGBT sentiment evokes anxiety and fear. In such climates, many have felt forced to keep their sexual desires and identity a secret, or to deny their same-sex sexual orientation due to a combination of powerful social and cultural influences (e.g. Rivers et al., 2010). In these oppressive environments extreme secrecy is necessary to avoid social and economic ostracism, and the possibility of criminal conviction (Barrett, 2008). It is perhaps not surprising that many studies, including that by Valentine and Waite (2012), found that individuals in these circumstances often develop identity conflicts.

Brennan-Ing et al. (2013), Barnes (2012),and Beagan (2014) found that individuals typically deal with these identity conflicts by doing one of the following: denying or rejecting their sexual identity, denying or rejecting their religious identity, integrating their identities, compartmentalising them or living with them.

Despite these struggles Brennan-Ing et al. found that many of these individuals in their study preferred to remain in their fundamentalist and conservative congregations despite the homonegativity they encountered (Walton, 2006; Pitt, 2010). Consequently, many LGBT individuals now continue to worship in their communities and local congregations where they regularly encounter homophobic attitudes and anti-gay rhetoric at odds with their sexual identities (Sherkat, 2002; Walton, 2006; Heerman et al., 2007; Pitt, 2010).

While there may be some commonality in terms of the life experiences (e.g. age, racism or homo/bi/transphobia), each 'other' identity added to this matrix (e.g. social class, disability, etc.) creates a new kaleidoscopic picture.

One way to conceptualise this multiplicity of identities and how they operate to create specific experiences is through intersectionality.

Intersectionality

Intersectionality, a term coined by Kimberlé Crenshaw in the late 1980s, has been variously conceptualised by authors, researchers and activists. According to Pheonix (2006), intersectionality describes "the complex political struggles and arguments that seek to make visible the multiple positioning that constitutes everyday life and the power relations that are central to it" (p. 187). Young and Meyer (2005) offer a comprehensive yet succinct description of intersectionality, stating that the key features of intersectionality are: (1) that no social group is homogeneous, (2) people must be located in terms of social structures that capture the power relations implied by those structures, and (3) there are unique, non-additive effects of identifying with more than one social group.

Exploring practices of intersectionality, Fisher (2003) suggests that the 'closet' is used as a space to 'negotiate the intersections of sexuality and ethnicity in everyday life' (p. 171). The 'micro-practices' she describes highlight the agility with which people who identify as belonging to multiple minority groups negotiate daily encounters, and also the skill required to balance uncomfortable, sometimes seemingly incompatible allegiances. We consider this in greater detail in the next section, drawing upon our own data as an illustrative case.

Our research study: identity formation and conflict in older Irish gay men

Our study[2] builds on previous research and examines the experiences of older Irish gay men, exploring the interaction between these identities and other significant identities, particularly religion. We explore the construction of gay identity and assess whether 'identity conflict' is an identifiable feature of the lives of our participants. Furthermore, we identify any sources of conflict and explore management and consequences of these conflicts.

Participants were recruited through poster advertisements in support agencies, on internet sites, in gay-identified venues and by 'snowballing'. The snowballing method was used to try to access men who did not access the 'gay scene'. The sample consisted of seven men, age range 56 to 68, all Irish nationals. We intentionally did not specify the lower age limit to participate in our study, but left it open for the participants to self-identify with the term 'older Irish gay men'. Three men lived in England and four in Ireland. All identified as 'gay'; however, only three identified as 'openly gay'. Four were single and three were in a relationship with a male partner (two of these participants were out). All men were of White Irish ethnicity. Five men grew up in a rural environment with two growing up in the city. All men identified as Catholics.

Interviews explored their experiences, perceptions and understanding of being an older gay person in Ireland and the UK (where some had migrated to), any concerns about that identity, and their views of the future. The interview followed a chronological sequence to capture experiences across the lifespan. Interviews were audio-recorded and transcribed verbatim by the first author (JM). We used thematic analysis (Braun and Clarke, 2006) to analyse the transcripts. This permitted us to explore data at both deductive and inductive levels. A naïve exploration of the data was completed, recording emergent codes and themes. Data were then reread, looking for instances related to Identity Process Theory (IPT), specifically: continuity, distinctiveness, self-efficacy and self-esteem. We employed a realist epistemological approach to theorise motivations, subjective experience and meaning. The critical lens further helps interrogate these phenomena by exploring (in)consistencies, contradictions and disunities in talk. This is significant because this study endeavours to enhance our understanding of the principles of identity when identity is perceived to be threatened. We found three themes from our data (Experiences of sexual awareness and identity conflict, 'Staying in' vs. 'Coming out', and Dealing with identity conflict). Each theme is discussed below, with anonymised quotes from our participants.

Experiences of sexual awareness and identity conflict

This theme addresses men's experiences of sexual awareness and identity acquisition, and the ensuing conflicts. Given the generally negative social representations associated with homosexuality in Ireland at the time of their youth, many men feared the prospect of discrimination and prejudice from their community if they revealed their sexual identities.

> There was an awful fear of discovery [...] negative to one's own identity. The feeling or, indeed, fear of who one is against the background of a straight version of society with feelings of confusion resulting in self-hate.
>
> (Eamon)

> Ireland, for me as a gay man, was bleak. It was a very bleak landscape and a very unforgiving landscape, and at the point of discovery or expression could be a very, very cruel landscape.
>
> (Brian)

This narrative of 'fear' and 'fear of discovery' has also been identified in other studies (see das Nair and Thomas, 2012). Due to the distinct heteronormative discourse that prevailed in Irish society at that time, men experienced sexual awareness in a very secretive manner, shrouded in shame. Participants feared the risk of association or affiliation with anything/one that was not 'straight'. Eamon, for instance said: "You are in a society where you are attracted to men not women and all the examples are male/female so it's incredibly confusing [having same-sex desires]." Indeed, some men reported feeling somewhat different from the 'norm' while growing up, and felt that they had neither the language nor awareness to identify or express these perceived anomalies.

Not having gay role models to identify with may have further exacerbated the men's sense of isolation, confusion and difference. Many described not even knowing the word 'homosexual':

> I think I was around 15 or 16 when I realised what the word homosexual even was. It was a total shock for me because I thought I was the only one.
>
> (Sam)

Situating these men in their youth where there was an absence of information, role models, or even the language to self-identify, acknowledge and articulate one's desires, sets the context in which they lived. Another major influence on this terrain was the Catholic Church, which wielded enormous power in Ireland at that time. Our participants described the influence of the Catholic Church as 'oppressive' and seeping into every aspect of society and daily life. There was a blurring of boundaries between religion and society, whereby religion was part and parcel of the culture itself. Eamon felt as though he were 'controlled' by the Church. This had a profound negative impact on his sense of self-efficacy:

> The Church was very, very, very powerful in Ireland at that time. And I think rather frighteningly powerful. The Church could absolutely destroy you. And if they destroyed you, they destroyed your family. The notion of maintaining one's respectability was very, very, strong.
>
> (Eamon)

It is interesting to note Eamon's concern not only for himself but for his family also. The idea of the Church being the grand patriarch of all people, who meted out edicts and punishments on them, was present in many of our participants' narratives. Due to this overwhelming power of the Church and the perceived threats of violating its codes of conduct, the participants described the task of trying to reconcile the religious and sexual facets of their lives, which were felt to be mutually incompatible, as being very difficult and isolating.

Most participants referred to the Church's negative outlook on homosexuality to explain and define their identity conflict. Fred explained: "I think the main issue wasn't my homosexuality it was the fact that it was against the law of the Church." This resonates with findings from Levy and Reeves' (2011) study which identified conflict between the Church's doctrine and same-sex attraction, which often left religious LGBT individuals feeling confused and fearful.

In our study, Bob saw his religion as being hypocritical:

> [W]e grew up in the 1940s and 1950s, and Ireland back then was crushed under the steamroller of the Vatican's hypocrisy. I mean, the hypocrisy was nauseating and that's how we all grew up, and it was a very repressive kind of upbringing.
>
> (Bob)

It is interesting to note the overlaps between our participants' experiences of the Catholic Church, and Haile and colleagues' (2011) and Woody's (2014, 2015) participants' experiences of the Black Church. In all these studies, the significance of a Church that coalesces under the banner of ethnicity (and thereby re-affirming ethnic and cultural identity) also disadvantages and excludes its members who are not seen as being heterosexual. Perhaps, it is for this reason that some of our participants had to carefully consider the merits of 'staying in' or 'coming out'.

'Staying in' versus 'Coming out'

This theme focused on both the nature of disclosure and non-disclosure of sexual identity to friends and family members, and the ensuing implications. Most men faced the conundrum of whether to disclose their sexual identity (to 'come out') or to keep it a secret from others (to 'stay in' or be 'closeted'). This included the challenge of 'staying in' or 'coming out' to themselves. Some participants reported that no one in their family or social network knew of their sexual identity, despite their own desire to disclose this information. Men used selective disclosure when speaking about their sexual identity, i.e. only telling people whom they felt would not react in a negative way: "I couldn't tell any of my friends as they were all straight. I met Irish men in gay bars and I could tell them, and that was alright, yeah" (Tom).

The coming-out process was lifelong, with some participants reporting that they were still not 'open' about their sexuality or were 'very guarded' about it. The reasons for not wanting to come out were myriad, with some finding self-disclosure or acceptance the first hurdle.

Furthermore, the management of information about sexual identity was difficult within small communities in Ireland, because of the close interrelations that defined them. Therefore, telling one person may have been tantamount to telling the town. Responses varied when participants disclosed their sexual orientation within family and peer groups, although most experienced some form of negative response. Religious-based family tensions and rejection was also a key theme in Westwood's study (2016).

Negative reactions, our participants felt, may have been due to a lack of others' understanding regarding sexuality. One misperception held by a family member was that sexuality was a personal desire and therefore could (and perhaps *should*) be ignored. The reaction that Tom got on disclosing his sexuality to his brother was: "I always knew you were selfish." The message is clear: sexuality is not solely an individual's issue, and therefore identifying as non-heterosexual (1) goes against the grain of society, and (2) causes distress to others. Other participants reported how people confused a gay identity with paedophilic interests and incestuous inclinations. This is reminiscent of one of Woody's (2014) participants' account of her in-laws not wanting to stay in her house because the in-laws had "two young daughters and I guess they thought we were going to jump them" (p. 152). The lack of knowledge evident in the culture regarding sexuality and the prevailing belief of the Church that homosexuality was indeed abnormal was evident in all our participants' narratives.

Those participants who encountered negative reactions to their disclosure of their sexuality disputed the right of others to judge them, which helped delegitimise others' views to a certain degree. This process decreased the threat to identity that negative views may have created (such as their potentially corrosive effect on self-esteem, or the attribution of negative distinctiveness to the person). Indeed, in the final theme from our study, we focus more on how people dealt with their identity conflicts.

Dealing with identity conflict

Our participants used various strategies to deal with their identity conflict. Most exercised extreme caution and discretion around their personal lives, keeping all aspects of their sexuality to themselves. Others developed divided lives – the 'straight life' during the day, and the 'gay life' by night.

Most participants spoke of how they had managed their religious and sexual identity by compartmentalising the Catholic and gay aspects of their lives. It was not so much that they tried to retain their 'Catholicism' or their 'gayness', but that they constantly felt that they were juggling two pre-existing and incompatible identities. Compartmentalisation is an intra-psychic strategy used to draw a strict boundary around the dissatisfying addition to the identity structure and therefore prevent the identity from being contaminated (Breakwell, 1986). Levy and Reeves' (2011) participants used the term 'compartmentalisation' to describe their efforts to keep sexual desires a secret. Compartmentalisation of aspects of the identity, however, can be an exhausting process, which can have detrimental effects on self-esteem. Fred reported the impact this had upon his life and his sense of well-being:

> When we go through something like that, no matter what it is, we often come out with scars, scars that will never heal, be it fear, be it a persecution complex, be it a feeling of inadequacy or difference, or whatever.
> (Fred)

Another coping mechanism used by some men was to differentiate between God's view on homosexuality and the Church's view on what it viewed as sexual deviance.

I'm conditioned now to see what I do as being wrong in the eyes of the Church and I say "in the eyes of the Church" as opposed to saying "in the eyes of God", because the eyes of the Church are looking at it in a specific way, and God looks at all of us in our total lives.

(Gordon)

Brennan-Ing (2013, p. 83) also found that older LGBT adults had a personal belief system which somewhat lessened the conflict between their religious and sexual identities. Participants in their study expressed a common theme as "a reliance on a personal spirituality that acknowledged an all-loving and all-inclusive God to whom homosexuality was not an issue".

Many participants backed away from the Church so that they could reconstruct their identities free from this judgement and guilt. They identified the prohibitive doctrine on homosexuality as a central threat to their gay identity. A remedy was to distance themselves from the Church. Some found this easier to do than others, since Catholicism often constituted more than just a religious identity. For some, their religion could be seen as a 'whole lifestyle', and therefore difficult to 'break free from'.

At one stage I decided to leave the Catholic Church and the battle with the guilt every Sunday was unbelievable, it was shocking to try and stop myself from going to Church or to find something else to do at that time.

(Eamon)

Other strategies for coping with identity conflict and threat involved participants reinterpreting and revising the context of their Catholic identity, thereby reducing the potential for conflict: "I still go to Church, yeah, I put their views to the back of my mind" (Tom).

Breakwell (1986) stated that individuals may attempt to separate the cohesion between incompatible aspects of their identity construction. This revision perhaps safeguards individuals' sense of continuity (as Catholics) and, therefore, offers a sense of coherence between sexual and religious identities. However, a subjective reconciliation between Catholicism and homosexuality was difficult and was still ongoing, without resolution, for some of our participants.

Participants responded to the historical context and culture in relation to their sexuality in different ways. While some managed to 'come out' without much difficulty, others kept their sexual identity hidden or suppressed. Participants who attempted to ensure that their sexuality was not disclosed within their communities used several strategies to achieve this. Again, parallels may be seen with Woody's (2014, 2015) participants' circumspection regarding coming out. Westwood (2016) also found this with many participants, especially the gay men, reporting that they had to try to lead heterosexual lives to avoid religious-based rejection from their families. Taylor (2011) also found that some participants interviewed said they make themselves 'ordinary' to fit in.

Some men distanced themselves from the 'gay scene' – almost adopting a heteronormative or 'straight-acting' stance at times. They kept their sexuality private and guarded against public display of sexual codes that could expose their sexuality. This interpersonal method of 'passing' may gain an individual social approval and contribute to self-esteem, thereby protecting the continuity of identity (Breakwell, 1986).

> I was always in the straight world, you know, and with straight friends, and we always went to the [straight] dance halls and bars and if you deviate and go somewhere else you would have to explain.
>
> (Tom)

This led to the apparent dismissal of those who did not act similarly: "Even nowadays, the flamboyant part, I was never into that, I never flaunted it" (Sam), and "I found them [effeminate men on the gay scene] very superficial" (Bob).

The similarity between these statements and those of some of Haile et al.'s (2011) participants is striking. One of their participants (Butch) said:

> It's the young queens [...] that make [...] the bad stigma for gay people. [...] They're just out of control [...] they wear scare drags [...] you know, they have on [...] girl pants, maybe a man's hat, with hair [...] they looking like a freak [...] and [...] that makes people look, that makes straight guys make comments.
>
> (Haile et al., 2011, p. 7)

By denigrating and distancing themselves from 'other (bad) gays' who were not like them, participants were able to incorporate their gay identity within a matrix of other conflicting identities, which helped reduce the tensions between identities.

These coping strategies seemed to enable some of our participants to disassociate 'doing gay things' (especially doing 'bad' gay things) from their self-concept and may have enhanced their self-esteem. However, it could also be construed as internalised homophobia towards feminine gay men or their mannerisms, and any overt demonstration of homosexuality (Reingardé, 2010). This internalised homophobia may then go on to delay the development of an authentic and integrated sexual orientation (Halkitis et al., 2009).

Some men employed the deflection strategy of identity denial to deal with the dilemma (Breakwell, 1986). Gordon's statement highlights this well: "Well, to be honest, I put it [same-sex sexuality] to the back of my mind and got on with life, you know, I wouldn't discuss it with anybody." This could perhaps be looked upon as a variation of the isolation strategy, often engaged when dealing with identity threat. Breakwell (1986) suggested that individuals may pull back from society in order to protect themselves from the risk of social rejection (of their sexual identity). The knock-on effect of this can be compromised self-esteem, as the individual emerges with a social distinction that is seen negatively. In these situations, people must create impermeable boundaries around the aspect of identity that is threatening. Thus, the gay aspect of their identity is kept separate from all other aspects of their identity. This method evolved as a problem-free philosophy of dealing with identity threat. Individuals could easily avoid identity conflict by shrouding an aspect of their identity.

Some participants responded to the negativity and discrimination surrounding their identity by emigrating. This was also reported in Levy and Reeves' study (2011) with participants moving to communities with resources for gay, lesbian and queer individuals where they had less difficulty resolving conflict. Indeed, in our study, many gay men disguised their real reason for leaving Ireland behind the need for employment and economic security. This culture of mass emigration gave men an excuse to leave Ireland and extricate themselves from repressive social and family environments. Their move from Ireland gave them a freedom and anonymity they had always craved. They were liberated in another land, finally able to live their lives as they chose.

Our study suggests that many gay Irish men faced challenges and barriers to constructing a stable gay identity, and for some this is ongoing. Religious and cultural experiences played a central role in Irish men's sexual identity acquisition and how they made sense of it. The results also demonstrated ways in which identity conflicts were created and how the men developed strategies to minimise these conflicts. In framing our analysis within an intersectional approach, we would endorse Brah's (1994) contention that such narratives must be seen against a historical, political, economic and cultural landscape that is constantly in flux. We see in our data how people connect with, struggle to connect with and actively distance themselves from the prevalent discourses; and the challenges they experience in negotiating the relationships between (and within) the self and society.

Discussion

Consistent with findings from existing research, we too found that most research has quite often been from the perspective of one identity characteristic (e.g. ethnicity and sexuality), but not more than one. Within the extant literature, being older, non-heterosexual and an ethnic minority or having a religious affiliation form specific sites of invisibility and we aimed to show in our research that it is possible to integrate multiple areas. Therefore, we set out to investigate research that would help us further understand the issues of LGBT people who identify as 'older' and as 'ethnic minority', and also to explore an additional identity (religion) and how these intersect.

In our review on ethnicity and older LGBT individuals we saw how multiple-minority statuses contributed to limitations or opportunities for older, non-heterosexual, ethnic minorities. We found concerns for men raised in the same religion (as the men in our study) but from different ethnic backgrounds (e.g. Latino men raised as Catholic showed high levels of internalised homophobia) (Halkitis et al., 2009). But there were also similar concerns for individuals not raised in a Catholic environment (e.g., David and Knight (2008) and Fredriksen-Goldsen and Muraco (2010) found many examples of individuals experiencing high levels of heteronormativity).

Consistent with findings from existing research on religion and older LGBT individuals the participants in our study tended to report similar identity conflicts when it comes to religiosity and sexuality. Furthermore they also reported similar ways of dealing with these conflicts.

With regard to ageing, Irish older gay men reported some ageism on the gay scene but not in everyday life, unlike African American older gay men (Woody, 2014). Woody's participants, like the participants in our study, spoke about a sense of alienation, feeling insignificant and feelings that their older age was seen as attracting yet another 'ism' (ageism) with which they had to contend. There is a sense of becoming invisible in some of the narratives, and a feeling of being isolated from their own ethnic communities but also from the wide LGBT society. However, it was apparent that as LGBT individuals aged they reported that they just want acceptance (in all areas of their lives). Fredriksen-Goldsen and Muraco's (2010) review also noticed the focus shift from dispelling the myth that older LGB people experience maladjusted ageing, to focusing on the psychosocial correlates of adjustment and functioning, to the social and community-based needs and experiences of older LGB people. Woody also reported on the resilience which LGBT individuals have developed with age, and the freedoms that ageing provides.

Conclusions

In concluding, we would like to go back to our premise of the invisibility or 'invisibilising' of older, ethnic minority, non-heterosexual people in the research literature – what Purdie-Vaughns and Eibach (2008) refer to as 'intersectional invisibility'. We believe there are many reasons for this invisibility. First, ageist stereotypes suggest that older people are non-sexual, and this is evident in the absences of sex and sexual health even in some policy documents published by the UK Department of Health (e.g. the National Service Framework for Older People and the National Sexual Health Strategy) (Bowman et al., 2006). Second, ethnic minorities are often not represented in research. The reasons for this may include: (1) researchers including but not describing their sample ethnically or coding their data along the lines of ethnicity; or (2) ethnic minorities not seeing themselves represented in the sample criteria set out or not aware of the importance that their contribution could make to research; or (3) researchers using exclusion criteria, such as excluding those for whom English is not their 'first language'.

Furthermore, while some ethnic minorities are stereotyped as being hypersexual, others are seen as being non-sexual (Han, 2005), thereby being missed out from research investigating LGBT issues. Therefore, what is needed is more engagement with ethnic minorities and for researchers to find acceptable ways in which people can be invited to take part in such research, perhaps through community leaders as channels to facilitate recruitment. Third, most research into non-heterosexuality relies on seeking people who identify as lesbian, gay, bisexual or trans. This, as demonstrated in research by Woody (2014, 2015) among others, is problematic because some ethnic minorities and perhaps some older people in general do not wish to label their sexuality or align themselves with the LGBT communities and their agenda. Therefore, it may be beneficial for sexuality research not to specify sexuality labels, or to use a range of more encompassing labels rather than relying solely on the 'LGBT' acronym. Finally, some older LGBT people who have a religious affiliation may seek to hide their sexuality or be discreet about it, thereby being missed out from general older LGBT research. Older, sexual minority, ethnic minority, with religious affiliations: each of these identities can create a new level or layer of invisibility.

Often, invisibility causes oppression, but for some older, ethnic minority, religious LGBT people, invisibility may offer respite from sexuality-based prejudice, allowing people to negotiate *how* to be read sexually:

> [W]e can walk down the street holding hands affectionately and kissing – without an eyebrow being raised because no one notices us – we have become invisible! We certainly do not regret the lack of reprisals. What is devastating is that with age we have become non-persons.
>
> (Grossman, 1997, p.17)

Invisibility can be a benefit for people, but only if they *choose* to be invisible when it suits them, not when it is imposed upon them. For researchers and policy makers, it is therefore imperative that we recognise our role in understanding this choice and to be mindful that we do not take this choice away.

Notes

1 We acknowledge that this is not a 'neutral' term either, and comes with its own problems.
2 A more thorough description of this study may be found in McCarthy (2013), unpublished Doctorate in Clinical Psychology thesis, submitted to the University of Lincoln, and McCarthy and das Nair (2017) 'Identity formation and conflict in older Irish gay men', *Psychology of Sexualities Review*, 8(1): 72–83.

References

Barnes, DM. and Meyer, IH. (2012) 'Religious affiliation, internalized homophobia, and mental health in lesbians, gay men, and bisexuals', *American Journal of Orthopsychiatry*, 82(4): 505–515.

Barrett, C. (2008). *A Project Exploring the Experiences of Gay, Lesbian, Bisexual, Transgender and Intersex Seniors in Aged-care Services*. Victoria: Matrix Gold.

Beagan, BL. and Hattie, B. (2014) 'LGBTQ experiences with religion and spirituality: Occupational transition and adaptation', *Journal of Occupational Science*, 22(4): 1–18.

Bowman, WP., Arcelus, J. and Benbow, SM. (2006) 'Nottingham study of sexuality & ageing (NoSSA I) – Attitudes regarding sexuality and older people: A review of the literature', *Sexual and Relationship Therapy*, 21(2): 149–161.

Brah, A. (1994) 'South Asian young Muslim women and the labour market', in Afshar, H. and Maynard, M. (eds), *The Dynamics of 'Race' and Gender: Some Feminist Interventions*. London: Taylor and Francis, pp. 151–171.

Braun, V. and Clarke, V. (2006) 'Using thematic analysis in psychology', *Qualitative Research in Psychology*, 3(2): 77–101.

Breakwell, GM. (1986). *Coping with Threatened Identities*. London and New York: Methuen.

Brennan-Ing, M., Seidel, L., Larson, B. and Karpiak, SE. (2013). '"I'm created in God's image, and God don't create junk": Religious participation and support among older GLBT adults', *Journal of Religion, Spirituality & Aging*, 25(2): 70–92.

das Nair, R. and Thomas, S. (2012) 'Religion', in das Nair, R. and Butler, C. (eds), *Intersectionality, Sexuality and Psychological Therapies: Working with Lesbian, Gay and Bisexual Diversity*. Chichester: BPS Blackwell, pp. 89–112.

David, S. and Knight, BG. (2008) 'Stress and coping among gay men: Age and ethnic differences', *Psychology and Aging*, 23(1): 62–69.

Fisher, D. (2003) 'Immigration closets: Tactical-micro-practices-in-the-hyphen', *Journal of Homosexuality*, 45(2/3/4): 171–192.

Fokkema, T. and Kuyper, L. (2009) 'The relation between social embeddedness and loneliness among older lesbian, gay, and bisexual adults in the Netherlands', *Archives of Sexual Behavior*, 38(2): 264–275.

Fredriksen-Goldsen, K. and Muraco, A. (2010) 'Aging and sexual orientation: A 25 year review of the literature', *Research on Aging*, 32(3): 372–413.

Grossman, AH. (1997) 'The virtual and actual identities of older lesbians and gay men', in Duberman, M. (ed.), *A Queer World: The Center for Lesbian and Gay Studies Reader*. New York: New York University Press, pp. 615–626.

Haile, R., Padilla, MB. and Parker, EA. (2011) '"Stuck in the quagmire of an HIV ghetto": The meaning of stigma in the lives of older black gay and bisexual men living with HIV in New York City Culture', *Health & Sexuality*, 13(4): 429–442.

Halkitis, P., Mattis, J., Sahadath, J., Massie, D., Ladyzhenskaya, L., Pitrelli, K. and Cowie, S. (2009) 'The meanings and manifestations of religion and spirituality among lesbian, gay, bisexual, and transgender adults', *Journal of Adult Development*, 16: 250–262.

Han, C-S. (2005) 'Gay Asian-American male seeks home', *The Gay & Lesbian Review Worldwide*. Available at www.glreview.org/article/article-1107/ (accessed 22 February 2016).

Hayman, S. (2011) 'Older people in Canada: Their victimization and fear of crime', *Canadian Journal on Aging/La Revue Canadienne du Vieillissement*, 30(3): 423–436.

Heerman, M., Wiggins, MI. and Rutter, PA. (2007) 'Creating a space for spiritual practice: Pastoral possibilities with sexual minorities', *Pastoral Psychology*, 55: 711–721.

Horner, B., McManus, A., Comfort, J., Freijah, R., Lovelock, G., Hunter, M. and Tavener, M. (2012) 'How prepared is the retirement and residential aged care sector in Western Australia for older non-heterosexual people?', *Quality in Primary Care,* 20(4): 263–274.

Jaspal, R. (2012) '"I never faced up to being gay": Sexual, religious and ethnic identities among British South Asian gay men', *Culture, Health and Sexuality: An International Journal for Research, Intervention and Care,* 14(7): 767–780.

Keogh, P., Henderson, L. and Dodds, C. (2004) *Ethnic Minority Gay Men. Redefining Community, Restoring Identity.* London: Sigma Research.

Levy, D. and Reeves, P. (2011) 'Resolving identity conflict: Gay, lesbian, and queer individuals with a Christian upbringing', *Journal of Gay & Lesbian Social Services,* 23(1): 53–68.

McCann, E., Sharek, D., Higgins, A., Sheerin, F. and Glacken, M. (2013) 'Lesbian, gay, bisexual and transgender older people in Ireland: Mental health issues', *Aging & Mental Health,* 17(3): 358–365.

Persson, DI. (2009) 'Unique challenges of transgender aging: Implications from the literature', *Journal of Gerontological Social Work,* 52(6): 633–646.

Pheonix, A. (2006) 'Editorial: Intersectionality', *European Journal of Women's Studies,* 13(3): 187–192.

Pitt, RN. (2010) '"Still looking for my Jonathan": Gay black men's management of religious and sexual identity conflicts', *Journal of Homosexuality,* 57(1): 39–53.

Porter, KE., Ronneberg, CR. and Witten, TM. (2013) 'Religious affiliation and successful aging among transgender older adults: Findings from the Trans MetLife Survey', *Journal of Religion, Spirituality & Aging,* 25(2): 112–138.

Purdie-Vaughns, V. and Eibach, RP. (2008) 'Intersectional invisibility: The distinctive advantages and disadvantages of multiple subordinate-group identities', *Sex Roles,* 59(5–6): 377–391.

Reingardė, J. (2010) 'Heteronormativity and silenced sexualities at work', *KultūralrVisuomenė,* 1(1): 83–96.

Rivers, I., McPherson, KE. and Hughes, JR. (2010) 'The role of social and professional support seeking in trauma recovery: Lesbian, gay and bisexual experiences of crime and fears for safety', *Psychology & Sexuality,* 1(2): 145–155.

Schnoor, RF. (2006) 'Being gay and Jewish: Negotiating intersecting identities', *Sociology of Religion,* 67(1): 43–60.

Sherkat, DE. (2002) 'Sexuality and religious commitment in the United States: An empirical examination', *Journal for the Scientific Study of Religion,* 41(2): 313–323.

Taylor, Y. (2011) 'Lesbian and gay parents' sexual citizenship: Costs of civic acceptance in the United Kingdom', *Gender, Place & Culture: A Journal of Feminist Geography,* 18(5): 583–601.

The Guardian. (2015) 'Is it time to ditch the term "black, Asian and minority ethnic" (BAME)?' Available at www.theguardian.com/commentisfree/2015/may/22/black-asian-minority-ethnic-bame-bme-trevor-phillips-racial-minorities (accessed 22 February 2016).

Valentine, G. and Waite, L. (2012) 'Negotiating difference through everyday encounters: The case of sexual orientation and religion and belief', *Antipode,* 44(2): 474–492.

Walton, G. (2006) '"Fag church": Men who integrate gay and Christian identities', *Journal of Homosexuality,* 51(2): 1–17.

Westerfield, EM. (2012) *Transgender Peoples' Experiences of Religion and Spirituality.* North Dakota State University.

Westwood, S. (2016) 'Religion, sexuality and (in)equality in the lives of older lesbian, gay and bisexual people in the UK', *Journal of Religion, Spirituality & Aging.* doi: 10.1080/15528030.2016.1155525.

Wintrip, S. (2009) *Not Safe For Us Yet: The Experiences and Views of Older Lesbian, Gay Men and Bisexuals Using Mental Health Services in London (A Scoping Study).* London: Polari Housing Association.

Witten, TM. (2015) 'Elder transgender lesbians: Exploring the intersection of age, lesbian sexual identity, and transgender identity', *Journal of Lesbian Studies,* 19(1): 73–89.

Woody, I. (2014) 'Aging out: A qualitative exploration of ageism and heterosexism among aging African American lesbians and gay men', *Journal of Homosexuality,* 61(1): 145–165.

Woody, I. (2015) 'Lift every voice: Voices of African-American lesbian elders', *Journal of Lesbian Studies,* 19(1): 50–58.

Young, R. and Meyer, I. (2005) 'The trouble with "MSM" and "WSW": Erasure of the sexual-minority person in public health discourse', *American Journal of Public Health,* 95(7): 1144–1149.

7   Gaps within gaps

Intersecting marginalisations of
older Black, Asian and minority
ethnic LGBT* people

Sue Westwood, Yiu-Tung Suen and Vernal Scott

Introduction

While there is a growing body of literature about lesbian, gay, bisexual
and trans* (LGBT*)[1] ageing, and about Black, Asian and minority ethnic
(BAME) ageing, with notable exceptions, very little has been published about
BAME and LGBT* people and ageing (Grossman, 2008; van Sluytman and
Torres, 2014; Gupta, 2015; Otis and Harley, 2016), particularly in the UK.
This chapter maps this knowledge gap by identifying and critically interrogating the absence of LGBT* voices from the literature on BAME ageing
and the absence of BAME voices from the literature on LGBT* ageing. It
then goes on to suggest what may be deduced about the experiences of ageing among BAME LGBT* people by overlaying the two respective sets of
literature on BAME and LGBT* ageing. The chapter then puts forward a
research agenda, identifying strategies which are needed to overcome barriers to LGBT* representation in BAME ageing research and barriers to
BAME representation in LGBT* ageing research.

Theoretical context

A central argument derived from reviewing the existing research literature in
the chapter is that BAME LGBT* people experience ageing differently from
White LGBT* older people and also from BAME older people. Their different experiences, we propose, are informed by the intersection of sexuality/
sexual identity and gender identity with 'race', culture, ethnicity (and religion), and the associated prejudices and discriminations throughout the
life course. Intersectionality was first introduced by Black feminist authors
Kimberlé Crenshaw (1991), bel hooks (1982) and Patricia Hill Collins (2000).
These authors showed how Black women experience sexism differently from
White women and racism differently from Black men, and argued that
Black women's experiences of prejudice and discrimination were informed
by the intersection of sexism and racism. Since then, intersectionality has
become a widely used framework to understand how inequalities work with

and through one another in ways which cannot be separated out (Taylor et al., 2011). Our interest in this chapter is in relation to how LGBT* and BAME social positions intersect (Bowleg, 2013) to inform the ageing experiences of older LGBT* people from BAME backgrounds, in addition to their intersections with other social positions.

A further argument in this chapter is about knowledge production, i.e. how knowledge about BAME/LGBT* ageing is produced, particularly in the context of academic research. The first key issue is a lack of intersectional theorising in relation to LGBT*/BAME ageing. As Julie Fish (2008) has argued, a failure to take an intersectional approach to LGBT* research has 'rendered the experiences of disabled, black and minority ethnic and other groups invisible and has contributed towards the homogenisation of LGBT* communities'. The second key issue relates to normativity in knowledge production. The work of the Black intersectionality theorists also informed the emergence of critical race theory (Tate, 2014). This provides a useful framework to develop understandings of the reproduction and consequences of institutional racism. A definition of institutional racism developed in the UK following the Macpherson inquiry on racial relations and the police force is set out as:

> The collective failure of an organisation to provide an appropriate and professional service to people because of their colour, culture, or ethnic origin. This can be seen or detected in processes, attitudes, and behaviour that amount to discrimination through unwitting prejudice, ignorance, thoughtlessness, and racist stereotyping which disadvantages people in ethnic minority groups.
>
> (Macpherson, 1999, para 6.34)

Institutional racism operates at the micro (individual attitudes and practices), macro (organisational) and meso (wider systemic) levels (Phillips, 2011). Since the early work of Patricia Hill Collins (2000), researchers have been highlighting the presence of institutional racism in academic contexts, both internationally and of relevance in this chapter, in the UK (Warmington, 2012). BAME staff in UK academia have self-reported 'experiences of invisibility, isolation, marginalisation and racial discrimination' in higher education (Equality Challenge Unit, 2009, p. 2). In addition, BAME lecturers teaching in the areas of 'race', equality and multiculturalism report that these subjects are often designated as 'low status' when performed by BAME staff, yet they appear to acquire higher status when performed by white staff. Overall, BAME staff report having fewer opportunities to develop research capacity and enhance their promotion prospects (Equality Challenge Unit, 2009, p. 2).

The comparative silence within UK academic research on LGBT* ageing that incorporates BAME issues may be attributed to institutionalised racism at micro, macro and meso levels. At the same time, there is a compelling argument to locate the comparative silence within UK academic research on BAME ageing about LGBT* issues within the context of prejudice and discrimination in relation to sexuality/sexual identity and/or gender identity. Heterosexism (the systematic privileging of heterosexual identities), heteronormativity (the assumption that heterosexuality is the norm), homophobia (prejudice and discrimination towards LG individuals) and biphobia (prejudice and discrimination towards bisexual individuals) are pervasive cultural phenomena, operating individually, collectively and systemically. Similarly, cisgenderism and sex/gender binarism operate on many levels, including institutionally:

> Cisgenderism refers to the cultural and systemic ideology that denies, denigrates, or pathologizes self-identified gender identities that do not align with assigned gender at birth as well as resulting behavior, expression, and community. This ideology endorses and perpetuates the belief that cisgender identities and expression are to be valued more than transgender identities and expression and creates an inherent system of associated power and privilege. The presence of cisgenderism exists in many cultural institutions, including language and the law, and consequently enables prejudice and discrimination against the transgender community.
>
> (Lennon and Mistler, 2014, p. 63)

Sex/gender binarism involves conceptually and discursively positioning people as either/or one of two genders, which is eluding for those individuals who mobilise fluid sex/gender identities. Both cisgenderism and sex/gender binarism in academia shape knowledge production, both in terms of what is thinkable and also what is researchable.

Background

Both LGBT* people and BAME people, and thus BAME LGBT* people, are part of the ageing population. The UK population is not only an ageing population; it is also becoming increasingly racially/ethnically diverse. It is projected that by 2051, the non-white ethnic minorities will have grown to 20.7 million, about 30 per cent of the total UK population. The largest ethnic minority group in 2051 will continue to be 'Other White', at 4 million, followed by the Indian (3.2 million), Black African (3 million), Pakistani (2.9 million), the diverse 'Other' group (1.7 million) and then the Bangladeshi, Mixed – White/Black Caribbean, Mixed – White/Asian and Chinese, each with 1.4 million (Lievesley, 2010, p. 54). This diversity is also reflected in the ageing population. It is estimated that by 2051 there will be 19 million people over the age of 65 in England and Wales (The Commons Library, 2010), of whom 3.8 million will be from BAME backgrounds (compared with 675,000 in 2010) (Lievesley, 2010, p 54).

There are no precise figures for the lesbian, gay, bisexual and trans* (LGBT*) populations, due partly to a lack of auditing (Aspinall, 2009) and also because they constitute a hidden community (Meyer and Wilson, 2009), in particular, still, among the trans* communities (Bailey, 2012). An esti-mated 7.5 to 10 per cent of the population identify as lesbian, gay and bisex-ual (LGB) (Aspinall, 2009; Knocker, 2012), although many consider this to be a significant underestimate (Coffman et al., 2013). Even based on these conservative figures, by 2051 there will be at least 1.4 million (7.5%) and 1.9 million (10%) LGB people aged over 65 in the UK, of whom at least be-tween 300,000 and 400,000 will be from BAME backgrounds. These figures are likely to be underestimations, since these populations are particularly hidden.

Despite this demographic, BAME LGBT* ageing is under-researched. UK gerontology is showing increasing interest in BAME ageing (e.g. Victor et al., 2012); however, this has not been paralleled by an interest in BAME LGBT* ageing. A US review of the literature on Black and African LGBT* people (of all ages) observed:

> One reason for this situation is the social stigma associated with LGBT* issues, both in Black and African American communities and in America in general. A second reason is that researchers have not gained entry, support, or trust in these communities. A third reason is the ex-tent to which investigators have considered research among Black and African American LGBT* persons unimportant.
>
> (Wheeler, 2003, p. 66)

The argument here is that the exclusion of LGBT* ageing from BAME dis-course is shaped by the norms and prejudices within which that discourse is located. Van Sluytman and Torres (2014) carried out a content analysis of the international literature on BAME LGBT* ageing (including 64 articles). They identified distinct cultural needs of sexual orientation and gender mi-norities but concluded that these populations remain underexplored. They further observed that BAME experiences were excluded in three main ways: in sampling in LGBT* studies which did not include a representative pro-portion of BAME people; in analyses which did not consider the dimensions of race and ethnicity; and in a lack of studies which focused specifically on LGBT* and BAME people. There is however a growing academic au-thorship from the USA and elsewhere specifically on BAME LGB ageing, including, for example, papers (to name but a few) on: vulnerability and resilience among African American older lesbians (e.g. Woody, 2015; Dibble et al., 2012); older Black lesbians and social justice (Battle et al., 2015); older Black lesbians living in rural areas (Harley et al., 2014); older Black gay and bisexual men living with HIV (Haile et al., 2011); 'racial disparities' in HIV and ageing (Linley et al., 2012); happiness and well-being among older Black gay men (Battle et al., 2013); and a study on ageism and heterosexism among older African American lesbians and gay men (Woody, 2014). In terms of other international authorship, Travis Kong's research on older gay men in Hong Kong stands out as a vanguard piece of work (Kong, 2012). There is also some grey literature on LGBT* ageing which includes race and ethnicity as a key or specific dimension (e.g. Espinoza, 2013, 2014). However, at the same time, some major reviews of USA academic authorship on LGBT* ageing (e.g. Fredriksen-Goldsen et al., 2013, 2014) have not included ethnicity as part of the sample demographics, but not analysed specific ethnic issues in the studies. Notably, however, the new US-based Handbook of LGBT* Elders (Harley and Tester, 2016) has multiple sections on BAME LGBT* ageing, such as African American and Black LGBT Elders, American Indian, Alaska Native, and Canadian Aboriginal Two-Spirit/LGBT Elderly and Asian American and Native Pacific Islander LGBT Elders, both adding to extant knowledge and also filling in many knowledge gaps in a US context.

Many older LGBT* people have been rejected by their families, and research from the USA suggests that the risk of rejection is greater among BAME communities (Hill, 2013). This is particularly an issue for those BAME LGBT* individuals whose families place a strong emphasis on traditional family ideals and gender norms (Kong, 2010) and/or hold strong religious beliefs. At the same time, older BAME LGB people are at risk of heightened exposure to racism within the LGB community (Han, 2008). These collective pieces of work suggest that older BAME LGB people may indeed find themselves excluded from both LGB and BAME communities at the intersection of racism, and homophobia, and transphobia (Harley, 2016), as well as being marginalised more broadly 'in a sexist, racist and ageist world' (Woody, 2015, p. 53). It is highly likely that bisexual people may feel further alienated within the lesbian and gay communities. While there is some authorship on younger African American trans* individuals (e.g. Stevens et al., 2013), there is little as yet on older African American trans* individuals.

In the UK, by contrast, authorship on BAME LGBT* ageing is scant. The first major UK study of LGB ageing was overwhelmingly 'white' (259, or 97.4%)' (Heaphy et al., 2004, p. 883), reflecting a general demographic in LGBT* ageing research, particularly in the UK (Clover, 2006).

The UK LGB (and recently also T) advocacy organisation, Stonewall, has produced reports on BAME issues. One report stated that while all LGB people (across the age spectrum) are more likely to be exposed to health risks (because of minority stress and by lifestyle, social exclusion and barriers to health screening), BAME LGB people are more likely to be exposed to those, and additional risks, and their consequences (Stonewall, 2012), meaning that they experience double jeopardy (i.e. disadvantage incurred from two sources simultaneously). For example, fewer Black than White lesbian and bisexual women said their health care professional had acknowledged that they were lesbian or bisexual after they had self-disclosed (p. 5); and a greater proportion of lesbian and bisexual women 'of mixed or other ethnicity' than

White lesbian and bisexual women had deliberately harmed themselves and/ or taken drugs during the previous year (p. 5). More Black than White gay and bisexual men had experienced domestic abuse from a family member since the age of 16 and greater numbers of White than BAME (sic) gay and bisexual men examine themselves for health checks (p. 7).

However, despite addressing BAME issues among younger LGB people, in Stonewall's report on the YouGov survey they commissioned (involving over 1,000 older lesbian, gay and bisexual people in the UK), the participant demographic was not analysed by ethnicity and BAME issues are not mentioned once in the entire document. In this way we can see how a lack of an intersectional approach can impede understandings of BAME LGBT* ageing.

Reporting on her difficulty in recruiting BAME participants to her UK research study of older LGB people, the White British author Sue Westwood argued that it is a demographic issue shaped by migration patterns in the 1950s and 1960s. There are currently many more older, White British people than older people with BAME identities in the United Kingdom, although this pattern will change as more recent migrants age (Westwood, 2013b, p. 386). She continued to speculate that 'race' plays an important part in the process of research production itself (Held, 2009): older BAME lesbians may be in different, and more complex, forms of hiding than older White lesbians; they may have social networks that deliberately, or by default, do not engage with White lesbian networks (Moore, 2006); they may be excluded by White networks through processes associated with racism (Davis, 2010); there may be a reluctance to have their stories 'captured' by a White researcher. Leela Bakshi has written: 'Me as a person of colour giving my story to be "processed" and "consumed" by a white researcher, uncomfortably reproduces the dynamics of colonialism' (in Bakshi and Traies, 2011, p. 2).

The Hong Kong author Suen (2015) also reported having made explicit efforts to reach BAME individuals in his research with older gay men in the UK, but encountered difficulties in persuading BAME LGBT* groups even just to convey information about his study to their group members. There is a need to better understand the reasons for these difficulties in engaging (older) BAME LGBT* people in research. There may be issues of identification. For example, a study of older African American lesbians and gay men in the USA (Battle et al., 2013) found that they showed an aversion to LGBT* labels because of the cultural connotations attached to the terms. This touches on the basic question whether LGBT* labels are applicable across cultures There are myriad social forces at work in shaping how individuals are defined and self-define themselves, and such decisions can be 'pragmatic, related to concerns of situational advantage, political gain, and conceptual utility' (Seidman, 1994, p. 173).

In the absence of a robust UK research base specifically on older BAME LGBT* ageing, we will now analyse UK research on BAME ageing and

LGBT* ageing respectively, and then consider what insights may be drawn from both in relation to older BAME LGBT* people.

Deductions from UK research on BAME older people and LGBT* older people

Research on older BAME people and on older LGBT* people in the UK would suggest that there are significant parallels in terms of later life inequalities. BAME older people are likely to be increasingly part of rural populations (Manthorpe et al., 2012) and may be at heightened risk of isolation and loneliness both as older people in rural areas and as BAME older people in rural areas. Older BAME people, partly those of South Asian origin, are more likely than White British older people to report limiting and poor self-rated health (Evandrou et al., 2015). Older people from BAME backgrounds tend to be less satisfied with social care provision than older people from White British backgrounds (R. Willis et al., 2016). They report concerns about 'the incomplete recognition of the culturally-specific needs of older people from black and minority ethnic groups by mainstream services' (Manthorpe et al., 2009, p. 109). In particular, care services are considered to lack competence in recognising and supporting cultural and ethnic diversity (Sharif et al., 2008; Badger et al., 2009; Desai, 2012), especially intersecting diversities. People from BAME backgrounds are less likely to die at home, more likely to die in hospital, and less likely to have access to hospice care than are White British people in the UK (Calanzani et al., 2014; Dixon et al., 2015).

Social policy appears ill-equipped to address the additional burdens placed on informal carers of older people in BAME cultures (Katbamna et al., 2004), especially where care of older people is considered to be a family duty and the need for formal support a 'failure' of the family (Bowes and Wilkinson, 2003). This is particularly the case for older BAME people with dementia (Moriarty et al., 2011; Osman and Carare, 2015). In terms of protecting older BAME people from elder abuse, Manthorpe and Bowes (2010, p. 263) have argued that they are under-protected compared with White British people and that there is 'a continuing separation of matters of race and ethnicity from mainstream policy and practice thinking. Safeguarding policies lack cultural competence and sensitivity.'

Research with older LGBT* people in the UK echoes many of the concerns of older BAME people. For example, social connectedness is a concern for older LGBT people that might overlap with concerns for older BAME people. Older LGBT people may be at heightened risk of isolation and loneliness (Heaphy, 2009). Older LGB people in the UK, compared with older heterosexual people (Guasp, 2011), are more likely to be single, to not have children and to be estranged from their biological families. Some (older) LGB people may experience exclusion from religious/faith groups (Westwood, 2017), particularly those from BAME backgrounds (Scott, 2013).

Such issues with social belonging are similar to what we know about BAME older people. Older LGBT people are more likely to take drugs, to have a history of mental illness and concerns about their mental health, particularly anxiety and depression (Guasp, 2011). The latter is associated with accumulated minority stress, i.e. lifelong effects of social marginalisation (Fredriksen-Goldsen et al., 2013). This may also be the case for older BAME people.

Older LGBT people are more likely to need formal care provision sooner and in disproportionate numbers to older heterosexual and cisgender people (Westwood et al., 2015). Reasons for this include a comparatively lower level of intergenerational support and heightened health and social care needs, Yet, at the same time, older LGBT* people in the UK have major concerns about health and social care provision which they perceive as being ill-equipped to recognise and meet their needs (Almack, 2010; Westwood, 2015; Westwood et al., 2015; Hunter et al., 2016). Guasp (2011) reported on a survey of older LGB people in the UK that:

> Nearly half would be uncomfortable being out to care home staff, a third would be uncomfortable being out to a housing provider, hospital staff or a paid carer, and one in five wouldn't feel comfortable disclosing their sexual orientation to their GP. Significant numbers of disabled lesbian, gay and bisexual people also report that they have not accessed the health, mental health and social care services in the last year that they felt they needed.
>
> (Guasp 2011, p. 3)

There is a lack of recognition of LGBT* carers in the UK (Hines, 2007; Willis et al., 2011), including those who are supporting older LGBT* people (Cronin et al., 2011), especially those with dementia (Price, 2016). This lack of recognition can lead, in turn, to a lack of appropriate carer support. UK community care policy is predicated upon notions of biological family and community support which may not necessarily reflect the social support networks of older LGBT* people, particularly those who have been rejected by their families and/or have geographically dispersed communities (Almack, 2010; Bailey, 2012; Westwood, 2013b). Limited research thus far would suggest that residential care provision is also under-prepared to recognise and/or meet the needs of older LGBT* people in the UK (Walker et al., 2013; P. Willis et al., 2016; Hafford-Letchfield et al., 2018). Palliative care services in particular are under-equipped to meet the needs of LGBT* people at end of life (Dixon et al., 2015; Almack and National Council for Palliative Care, 2016).

In terms of protecting older LGBT* people from elder abuse, while links have been made between LGBT* ageing and elder abuse in the USA (Cook-Daniels, 1998), there have been less explicit connections in the UK. Ward et al. (2010) have raised equality and human rights concerns with regard to social care provision for older LGB people. In addition, West-wood (2016) has argued that, given that discriminatory abuse is defined in UK safeguarding policy as a form of elder abuse (Department of Health, 2000, Section 2.7), then any time an older/very old LGBT* person is exposed to homophobic and/or bi/transphobic abuse, they are encountering 'elder abuse'.

While the studies above have been mainly based on findings with older White LGBT* people, it may be argued that older BAME LGBT* people are at increased risk of many intersecting inequalities, including: loneliness and isolation, especially for those living in rural areas; health inequalities, including those associated with a lifetime of marginalisation; and health and social care inequalities in the form of services which are not equipped to respond to diversity among older people, especially intersecting diversities. An added aspect of inequality for older BAME LGBT* people relates to informal social support. This would suggest that older BAME LGBT* people are at increased risk of inadequate social support compared with older White British LGBT* people and older BAME heterosexual and/or cisgender people. They are also at heightened risk of elder abuse in the form of both BAME and LGBT* discriminatory abuse. It is also possible that older BAME LGBT* people have acquired specific multiple sets of skills to manage marginalisation (e.g. Berger, 1996); however, there is a need for research to explore this possibility.

The marginalisation in knowledge of and understanding about BAME LGBT* ageing will also have a knock-on effect for services. This is high-lighted in a recent chapter on improving health and social care provision for older LGBT* people which included a hypothetical scenario about a 70-year-old British gay man of African Caribbean descent with dementia. (Westwood et al., 2015). Clearly such gaps in knowledge (and support) need to be addressed as a matter of urgency.

Setting and implementing a research agenda

On the one hand, setting a research agenda is fairly simple. In order to ad-dress the gaps in knowledge about BAME LGBT* ageing, particularly in the UK, the following needs to occur:

1   Inclusive sampling and research strategies are essential (Van Sluytman and Torres, 2014, pp. 145–146). Mainstream sampling in ageing research should include purposive sampling to ensure that ageing diversity is ap-propriately represented.
2   Ageing research teams should ensure that they themselves reflect diver-sity, including BAME and LGBT* diversity, and they should also en-sure that their advisory groups do so too. This is particularly important when research teams themselves are not representative of population diversity.

3   All dissemination of ageing research should be clear, from the outset, about the extent to which samples on which empirical research is based do/do not represent heterogeneity of the ageing population. Specifically, existing research on LGBT* ageing which does not consider BAME ageing, and research on BAME ageing which does not consider LGBT* ageing needs to be approached with those conceptual/sampling limitations in mind (Otis and Harley, 2016).
4   Ageing research should use an intersectionality framework to understand how different social positions interact with one another to inform ageing experiences and later life outcomes: 'the use of an intersectional lens is critical' (Van Sluytman and Torres, 2014, p. 149).
5   With specific regard to BAME ageing research, such an intersectional approach would require including the perspectives of BAME older people from a wide range of social positions, including BAME LGBT* older people.
6   With specific regard to LGBT* ageing research, such an intersectional approach would require including the perspectives of LGBT* older people from a wide range of social positions, including BAME LGBT* older people.

Implementing such a research agenda is more complex. Many White British researchers have highlighted the 'difficulties' of accessing 'hard-to-reach' populations, including BAME populations. In this case, the privileged majority are White British LGBT* people in terms of LGBT* research, and heterosexual and/or cisgender BAME people in term of BAME research. How privileged academic researchers reach and represent the voices of 'hidden populations' has vexed researchers and filled research ethics journals for many years. There are tensions between wanting to facilitate the hearing of those marginalised voices, and privileged researchers not wanting to appropriate them for their own career advancement. When the researchers are White British and the 'hidden population' are BAME individuals, colonialism is quickly evoked (Allan and Westwood, 2015). Yet the answer is not simply that White British researchers leave the issue to BAME researchers, not least because of the marginalisation of BAME academics, particularly in the UK. There is also the issue of the unfairness of positioning marginalised individuals as the experts in their own and others' marginalisation. A way forward is to develop collaborative working on many levels. Writing in the USA, Wheeler advises:

> First, critical self-assessment is a necessity when conducting research on Black and African American LGBT* populations. Second, researchers must develop partnerships with members of the community from the outset of the enterprise. Third, investigators must develop cogent ways of reaching the populations of interest. Fourth, researchers must develop appropriate instrumentation. Finally, dissemination

of the findings should be handled collaboratively with members of the community.

(Wheeler, 2003, pp. 76–77)

Writing in the UK, Manthorpe and colleagues have argued for the need:

> To use multiple routes to encourage participation from minority groups, to seek the assistance of black and minority voluntary and community organisations as well as general older people's organisations, and to use well-tried methods of public engagement and public consultation. These methods pay attention to details of access, reimbursement and friendliness. [...] Black and minority ethnic older citizens are not always hard to reach or hard to hear, particularly where a rich civil society is engaged in the consultation processes.
>
> (Manthorpe et al., 2009, p. 109)

Specifically, Westwood (2013b) has argued elsewhere for the need for Participatory Action Research: 'with PAR the researched become co-researchers, giving them power and control over what knowledge is produced, as well as how that knowledge is deployed' (p. 389). Most important of all is approaching research with an emancipatory agenda, with the goals of: inclusivity, representation of diversity and heterogeneity, and analyses of intersecting (in)equalities.

Conclusion

This chapter has outlined the considerable gaps in knowledge about BAME LGBT* ageing, particularly in the UK. It has considered some of the reasons for those gaps. Drawing upon older BAME research and older LGBT* research respectively, it has suggested areas of in/exclusion which may intersect to produce and compound marginalisation encountered by BAME LGBT* people in later life. There is great need for research in this area, and we have outlined a possible research agenda. Such an agenda must of course be defined by older BAME LGBT* people themselves. They should also be central to and active participants in every aspect of the research process about older BAME LGBT* lives, particularly in terms of recruitment, data collection, analysis, and most importantly the dissemination of findings. It is essential that the voices of older BAME LGBT* people are not only heard, but that they also retain control of their stories and how they are heard.

Note

1 Trans* is an umbrella term which covers the gender identity spectrum: including (but not limited to) transgender, transsexual, transvestite, genderqueer, gender-fluid, non-binary, genderless, agender, non-gendered, third gender, two-spirit and bigender (Tompkins, 2014).

References

Allan, H. and Westwood, S. (2015) 'White British researchers and internationally educated research participants: Insights from reflective practices on issues of language and culture in nursing contexts', *Journal of Research in Nursing,* 20(8): 640–652.

Almack, K. and National Council of Palliative Care (2016) *Being Accepted Being Me: Understanding the End of Life Care Needs for Older LGBT People.* London: NCPC.

Aspinall, P. (2009). *Estimating the Size and Composition of the Lesbian, Gay, and Bisexual Population in Britain.* London: Equality and Human Rights Commission.

Badger, F., Pumphrey, R., Clarke, L., Clifford, C., Gill, P., Greenfield, S. and Knight Jackson, A. (2009) 'The role of ethnicity in end-of-life care in care homes for older people in the UK: A literature review', *Diversity in Health and Care,* 6(1): 23–29.

Bailey, L. (2012). 'Trans ageing', in Ward, R., Rivers, I. and Sutherland, M. (eds), *Lesbian, Gay, Bisexual and Transgender Ageing: Biographical Approaches for Inclusive Care and Support.* London; Philadelphia, PA: Jessica Kingsley, pp. 51–66.

Bakshi, L. and Traies, J. (2011) '"Come out, come out, wherever you are": The problem of representativeness and BME "participation" in LGBT/lesbian research.' A dialogue presented at the eighteenth *Lesbian Lives Conference,* University of Brighton, 12 February.

Battle, J., Daniels, J. and Pastrana Jr, AJ. (2015) 'Civic engagement, religion, and health: Older Black lesbians in the Social Justice Sexuality (SJS) Survey', *Women, Gender, and Families of Color,* 3(1): 19–35.

Battle, J., Daniels, J., Antonio, P., Turner, CB. and Eespinoza, A. (2013) 'Never too old to feel good: Happiness and health among a national sample of older Black gay men', *Spectrum: A Journal on Black Men,* 2(1): 1–18.

Berger, R. (1996) *Gay and Gray: The Older Homosexual Man, Second Edition.* New York: Routledge.

Bowes, A. and Wilkinson, H. (2003) '"We didn't know it would get that bad": South Asian experiences of dementia and the service response', *Health and Social Care in the Community,* 11(5): 387–396.

Bowleg, L. (2013). '"Once you've blended the cake, you can't take the parts back to the main ingredients": Black gay and bisexual men's descriptions and experiences of intersectionality', *Sex Roles,* 68(11–12): 754–767.

Calanzani, N., Koffman, J. and Higginson, I. (2014) *Palliative and End of Life for Black, Asian and Minority Ethnic Groups in the UK: Demographic Profile and the Current State of Palliative and End of Life Care Provision.* London: King's College London, Cicely Saunders Institute and Public Health England.

Clover, D. (2006) 'Overcoming barriers for older gay men in the use of health services: A qualitative study of growing older, sexuality and health', *Health Education Journal,* 65(1): 41–52.

Coffman, KB., Coffman, LC. and Ericson, KMM. (2013) The size of the LGBT* population and the magnitude of anti-gay sentiment are substantially underestimated. No. w19508. National Bureau of Economic Research. Available at http://bit.ly/1r40fXB (accessed 11 December 2014).

Collins, P. Hill (2000). *Black Feminist Thought: Knowledge, Consciousness and the Politics of Empowerment. Second Edition.* London: Routledge.

Cook-Daniels, L. (1998) 'Lesbian, gay male, bisexual and transgendered elders: Elder abuse and neglect issues', *Journal of Elder Abuse & Neglect,* 9(2): 35–49.

Crenshaw, K. (1991) 'Mapping the margins: Intersectionality, identity politics, and violence against women of color', *Stanford Law Review,* 43(6): 1241–1299.

Cronin, A. (2006). 'Sexuality in gerontology: A heteronormative presence, a queer absence', in Daatland DO. and Biggs, S. (eds), *Ageing and Diversity: Multiple Pathways & Cultural Migrations.* Bristol: Policy Press, pp. 107–122.

Cronin, A., Ward, R., Pugh, S., King, A. and Price, E. (2011) 'Categories and their consequences: Understanding and supporting the caring relationships of older lesbian, gay and bisexual people', *International Social Work,* 54(3): 421–435.

Davis, K. (2010) 'Avoiding the 'R-word': Racism in feminist collectives', in Ryan-Flood, R. and Gill, R. (eds), *Secrets and Silences in the Research Process.* London: Routledge, pp. 148–160.

Department of Health (2000). *No Secrets: Guidance on Developing and Implementing Multi-agency Policies and Procedures to Protect Vulnerable Adults from Abuse.* London: The Stationery Office.

Desai, S. (2012) 'Will it ever change? The continuing unmet needs of older black and ethnic minority people and social care', *Diversity and Equality in Health and Care,* 9: 85–87.

Dibble, SL., Eliason, MJ. and Crawford, B. (2012) 'Correlates of wellbeing among African American lesbians', *Journal of Homosexuality,* 59(6): 820–838.

Dixon, J., King, D., Matosevic, T., Clark, M. and Knapp, M. (2015). *Equity in the Provision of Palliative Care in the UK: Review of Evidence.* London: Personal Social Services Research Unit, London School of Economics and Political Science.

Equality Challenge Unit (2009) *The Experience of Black and Minority Ethnic Staff Working in Higher Education: Literature Review 2009.* London: Equality Challenge Unit.

Espinoza, R. (2013) *Health Equity & LGBT* Elders of Color.* New York: Services and Advocacy for GLBT Elders (SAGE).

Espinoza, R. (2014) *Out & Visible: The Experiences and Attitudes of LGBT* Older Adults, Ages 45–75.* New York: Services and Advocacy for GLBT Elders (SAGE).

Evandrou, M., Falkingham, J., Feng, Z. and Vlachantoni, A. (2015) *Two Decades On: The Continuing Health Disadvantage of South Asian Elders.* ESRC Centre for Population Change, June 2015. London: ESRC.

Fish, J. (2008) 'Navigating Queer Street: Researching the intersections of lesbian, gay, bisexual and trans (LGBT*Q) identities in health research', *Sociological Research Online,* 13(1). Available at www.socresonline.org.uk/13/1/12 (accessed 29 October 2015).

Fredriksen-Goldsen, KI., Cook-Daniels, L., Kim, HJ., Erosheva, EA., Emlet, CA., Hoy-Ellis, CP. and Muraco, A. (2014) 'Physical and mental health of transgender older adults: An at-risk and underserved population', *The Gerontologist,* 54(3): 488–500.

Fredriksen-Goldsen, KI., Emlet, CA., Kim, HJ., Muraco, A., Erosheva, EA., Goldsen, J. and Hoy-Ellis, CP. (2013) 'The physical and mental health of lesbian, gay male, and bisexual (LGB) older adults: The role of key health indicators and risk and protective factors', *The Gerontologist,* 53(4): 664–675.

Grossman, A. (2008). 'Conducting research among older lesbian, gay and bisexual adults', *Journal of Gay and Lesbian Social Services,* 20: 51–67.

Guasp, A. (2011). *Lesbian, Gay and Bisexual People in Later Life.* London: Stonewall.

Gupta, K. (2015) Where are our elders? [Online] 29 January 2015. Available at http://mixosaurus.co.uk/2015/01/where-are-our-elders-2/ (accessed 29 October 2015).

Hafford-Letchfield, T., Willis, P., Almack, K. and Simpson, P. (2018) 'Developing inclusive residential care for older Lesbian, Gay, Bisexual and Trans (LGBT) people: An evaluation of the Care Home Challenge action research project', *Health and Social Care in the Community*, 26(2): 312–320.

Haile, R., Padilla, MB. and Parker, EA. (2011) '"Stuck in the quagmire of an HIV ghetto": The meaning of stigma in the lives of older black gay and bisexual men living with HIV in New York City', *Culture, Health & Sexuality*, 13(4): 429–442.

Han, CS. (2008) 'They don't want to cruise your type: Gay men of color and the racial politics of exclusion', *Social Identities: Journal for the Study of Race, Nation and Culture,* 13(1): 51–67.

Harley, DA. (2016) 'African-American and Black LGBT* elders', in Harley, DA. and Teaster, PB. (eds), *Handbook of LGBT* Elders*. New York; London: Springer, pp. 105–134.

Harley, DA. and Teaster, PB. (eds) (2015) *Handbook of LGBT* Elders*. New York; London: Springer.

Harley, DA., Stansbury, KL., Nelson, M. and Espinosa, CT. (2014) 'A profile of rural African American lesbian elders: Meeting their needs', in Ofahengaue Vakalahi, HF., Simpson, GM. and Giunta, N. (eds), *The Collective Spirit of Aging Across Cultures*. New York: Springer, pp. 133–155.

Heaphy, B. (2009) 'The storied, complex lives of older GLBT adults; Choice and its limits in older lesbian and gay narratives of relational life', *Journal of GLBT Family Studies*, 5: 119–138.

Heaphy, B., Yip, A. and Thompson, D. (2004) 'Ageing in a non-heterosexual context', *Ageing & Society*, 24(6): 881–902.

Held, N. (2009) 'Researching "race" in lesbian space: A critical reflection', *Journal of Lesbian Studies*, 13(2): 204–215.

Herek, G. (2004) 'Beyond "homophobia": Thinking about sexual prejudice and stigma in the twenty-first century', *Sexuality Research and Social Policy*, 1(2): 6–24.

Hill, MJ. (2013) 'Is the Black community more homophobic? Reflections on the intersectionality of race, class, gender, culture and religiosity of the perception of homophobia in the Black community', *Journal of Gay & Lesbian Mental Health*, 17(2): 208–214.

Hines, S. (2007) 'Transgendering care: Practices of care within transgender communities', *Critical Social Policy*, 27(4): 462–486.

hooks, bel (1982) *Ain't I a Woman: Black Women and Feminism*. London: Pluto.

Hunter, C., Bishop, J-A. and Westwood, S. (2016) 'The complexity of trans*/gender identities: Implications for dementia care', in Westwood, S. and Price, E. (eds), *Lesbian, Gay, Bisexual and Transgender (LGBT*) Individuals Living with Dementia: Concepts, Practice and Rights*. Abingdon: Routledge, pp. 124–137.

Katbamna, S., Ahmad, W., Bhakta, P., Baker, R. and Parker, G. (2004) 'Do they look after their own? Informal support for South Asian carers', *Health & Social Care in the Community*, 12(5): 398–406.

Knocker, S. (2012) *Perspectives on Ageing Lesbians, Gay Men and Bisexuals*. London: Joseph Rowntree Foundation.

Kong, TSK. (2010) *Chinese Male Homosexualities: Memba, Tongzhi and Golden Boy*. London: Routledge.

Kong, TSK. (2012) 'A fading Tongzhi heterotopia: Hong Kong older gay men's use of spaces', *Sexualities*, 15(8): 896–916.

Lennon, E. and Mistler, BJ. (2014) 'Cisgenderism', *TSQ: Transgender Studies Quarterly*, 1(1–2): 63–64.

Lievesley, N. (2010). *The Future Ageing of the Ethnic Minority Population of England and Wales*. London: Centre for Policy on Ageing (CPA).

Linley, L., Prejean, J., An, Q., Chen, M. and Hall, HI. (2012) 'Racial/ethnic disparities in HIV diagnoses among persons aged 50 years and older in 37 US states, 2005–2008', *American Journal of Public Health*, 102(8): 1527–1534.

Macpherson W. (1999) *The Stephen Lawrence Inquiry. Report of an Inquiry by Sir William Macpherson of Cluny*. London: Stationery Office.

Manthorpe, J. and Bowes, A. (2010) 'Age, ethnicity and equalities: Synthesising policy and practice messages from two recent studies of elder abuse in the UK', *Social Policy and Society*, 9(2): 255–265.

Manthorpe, J., Iliffe, S., Moriarty, J., Cornes, M., Clough, R., Bright, L. and Rapaport, J. (2009) '"We are not blaming anyone, but if we don't know about amenities, we cannot seek them out": Black and minority older people's views on the quality of local health and personal social services in England', Ageing *and Society*, 29(1): 93–113.

Meyer, H and Wilson, PA. (2009) Sampling Lesbian, Gay, and Bisexual Populations. *Journal of Counseling Psychology, American Psychological Association*, 56(1): 23–31.

Moore, M. (2006) 'Lipstick or Timberlands? Meanings of gender representation in Black lesbian communities', *Signs: Journal of Women in Culture and Society*, 32(1): 113–139.

Moriarty, J., Sharif, N. and Robinson, J. (2011) *Black and Minority Ethnic People with Dementia and their Access to Support and Services*. London: Social Care Institute for Excellence.

National Council for Palliative Care (NCPC) (2012) *The Route to Success in End of Life Care – Achieving Quality for Lesbian, Gay, Bisexual and Transgender People*. London: NCPC.

Osman, S. and Carare, RO. (2015) 'Barriers faced by the people with dementia in the Black and Minority Ethnic groups in accessing health care and social services', *Journal of Gerontology & Geriatric Research*, http://dx.doi.org/10.4172/2167-7182.1000198.

Otis, MD. and Harley, DA. (2016) 'The intersection of identities of LGBT* elders: Race, age, sexuality, and care network', in Harley, DA. and Teaster, PB. (eds), *Handbook of LGBT* Elders*. New York: Springer, pp. 83–101.

Phillips, C. (2011) 'Institutional racism and ethnic inequalities: An expanded multilevel framework', *Journal of Social Policy*, 40(1): 173–192.

Price, E. (2016) 'Looking back whilst moving forward: LGBT** carers' perspectives', in Westwood, S. and Price, E. (eds), *Lesbian, Gay, Bisexual and Transgender (LGBT*) Individuals Living with Dementia: Concepts, Practice and Rights*. Abingdon: Routledge, pp. 138–154.

Scott, V. (2013) *God's Other Children*. CreateSpace Independent Publishing Platform.

Seidman, S. (1994) 'Queer-ing sociology, sociologizing queer theory: An introduction', *Sociological Theory*, 12: 166–177.

Sharif, N., Brown, W. and Rutter, D. (2008) *The Extent and Impact of Depression on BME Older People and the Acceptability, Accessibility and Effectiveness of Social Care Provision*. London: Social Care Institute for Excellence (SCIE).

Stevens, R., Bernadini, S. and Jemmott, JB. (2013) 'Social environment and sexual risk-taking among gay and transgender African American youth', *Culture, Health & Sexuality*, 15(10): 1148–1161.

Stonewall (2012) *Ethnicity: Stonewall Health Briefing*. London: Stonewall.

Suen, Y-T. (2015) 'What's gay about being single? A qualitative study of the lived experiences of older single gay men', *Sociological Research Online*, 20(3): 1–7.

Tate, SA. (2014) '"I can't quite put my finger on it": Racism's touch', *Ethnicities*, 16(1): 68–85.

Taylor, Y., Hines, S. and Casey, M. (eds) (2011) *Theorizing Intersectionality and Sexuality*. Basingstoke: Palgrave Macmillan.

The Commons Library (2010) *The Ageing Population: Key Issues for the 2010 Parliament*. London: HM Government. Available at www.parliament.uk/business/publications/research/key-issues-for-the-new-parliament/value-for-money-in-public-services/the-ageing-population/.

Tompkins, A. (2014) 'Asterisk', *TSQ: Transgender Studies Quarterly*, 1(1–2): 26–27.

Van Sluytman, LG. and Torres, D. (2014) 'Hidden or uninvited? A content analysis of elder LGBT* of color literature in gerontology', Journal *of Gerontological Social Work*, 57(2–4): 130–160.

Victor, CR., Burholt, V. and Martin, W. (2012) 'Loneliness and ethnic minority elders in Great Britain: An exploratory study', *Journal of Cross-cultural Gerontology*, 27(1): 65–78.

Walker, R., Hughes, C., Ives, D. and Jardine, Y. (2013). *Assessment of Care Needs and the Delivery of Care to Older Lesbians Living in Residential Care Homes in Bradford and Calderdale*. Bradford: The Labrys Trust.

Ward, R., Pugh, S. and Price, E. (2010) *Don't Look Back? Improving Health and Social Care Service Delivery for Older LGB Users*. Manchester: Equality and Human Rights Commission.

Warmington, P. (2012) '"A tradition in ceaseless motion": Critical race theory and black British intellectual spaces', *Race Ethnicity and Education*, 15(1): 5–21.

Weeks, J. (2000). *Making Sexual History*. Cambridge: Polity Press.

Westwood, S. (2013a) '"My friends are my family": An argument about the limitations of contemporary law's recognition of relationships in later life', *Journal of Social Welfare & Family Law,* 35(3): 347–363.

Westwood, S. (2013b) 'Researching older lesbians: Problems and partial solutions', *Journal of Lesbian Studies*, 17(3–4): 380–392.

Westwood, S. (2015) '"We see it as being heterosexualised, being put into a care home": Gender, sexuality and housing/care preferences among older LGB individuals in the UK', *Health and Social Care in the Community*. doi: 10.1111/hsc.12265.

Westwood, S. (2016) Ageing, Gender and Sexuality: Equality in Later Life. London: Routledge.

Westwood, S. (2017) 'Religion, sexuality and (in)equality in the lives of older lesbian, gay and bisexual people in the UK', *Journal of Religion, Spirituality & Ageing,* 29(1): 47–69.

Westwood, S., King, A., Almack, K., Suen, Y-T. and Bailey, L. (2015) Good practice in health and social care provision for older LGBT* people', in Fish, J. and Karban, K. (eds), *Social Work and Lesbian, Gay, Bisexual and Trans Health Inequalities: International Perspectives*. Bristol: Policy Press, pp. 145–159.

Wheeler, DP. (2003) 'Methodological issues in conducting community-based health and social services research among urban Black and African American LGBT* populations', *Journal of Gay & Lesbian Social Services*, 15(1–2): 65–78.

Willis, P., Ward, N. and Fish, J. (2011) 'Searching for LGBT* carers: Mapping a research agenda in social work and social care', *British Journal of Social Work*, 41(7): 1304–1320.

Willis, P., Maegusuku-Hewett, T., Raithby, M. and Miles, P. (2016) 'Swimming up-stream: The provision of inclusive care to older lesbian, gay and bisexual (LGB) adults in residential and nursing environments in Wales', *Ageing & Society,* 36(2): 282–306.

Willis, R., Khambhaita, P., Pathak, P. and Evandrou, M. (2016) 'Satisfaction with social care services among South Asian and White British older people: The need to understand the system', *Ageing and Society*, 36(7): 1364–1387.

Witten, TM. (2014) 'End of life, chronic illness, and trans-identities,' *Journal of Social Work in End-of-Life & Palliative Care*, 10(1): 34–58.

Witten, TM. (2016) 'Trans* people anticipating dementia care: Findings from the Transgender MetLife Survey', in Westwood, S. and Price, E. (eds), *Lesbian, Gay, Bisexual and Transgender (LGBT*) Individuals Living with Dementia: Concepts, Practice and Rights*. Abingdon: Routledge, pp. 110–123.

Woody, I. (2014) 'Aging out: A qualitative exploration of ageism and heterosexism among aging African American lesbians and gay men', *Journal of homosexuality*, 61(1): 145–165.

Woody, I. (2015) 'Lift every voice: Voices of African-American lesbian elders', *Journal of Lesbian Studies*, 19(1): 50–58.

8 Intergenerationality and LGBT ageing

Assessing the UK evidence base and its implications for policy

Dylan Kneale

Introduction

Intergenerational relationships span across living generations, extending beyond kinship relations to broader social networks, communities and societal solidarity. Familial intergenerational relationships are important conduits for the transmission of economic, social and cultural capital (Izuhara, 2010). However, transfer of capital between the generations is neither unidirectional nor confined to families alone. Intergenerational relations are an important dimension of the context in which people age. They: help to compose aspects of individuals' own social identity; can be important in enabling individuals to conceptualise and reconceptualise some of their own roles and identities; are important in moderating levels of citizenship and reciprocity; and, where focused on a particular goal or outcome, strong intergenerational relationships can help realise this (Kaplan, 1997; Reczek, 2014).

Among Lesbian, Gay, Bisexual and Transgender (LGBT) people, the nature of family and social networks is known to differ, and kinship networks may be in equal standing to relationships within 'families of choice' (Hughes and Kentlyn, 2011) and broader social networks. Alternative conceptualisations of 'family' may mean that establishing community-level intergenerational relationships holds added significance among LGBT people than for non-LGBT people, although LGBT spaces are often not naturally conducive for the development of intergenerational solidarity (Simpson, 2013). In this chapter the evidence base for, and progress in the development of, interventions to support and enhance intergenerational relations among LGBT people in the UK is critically explored.

The chapter begins with (1) a description of three innovative intergenerational LGBT projects and the supporting evidence base that existed; before (2) exploring new opportunities for quantitative research to enhance the evidence of need for intergenerational work among LGBT people in the UK and presenting the results from one such analysis; and concluding with (3) an exploration of how the evidence base for intergenerational work among LGBT people has developed since 2010/2011.

Innovations in UK intergenerational projects for LGBT people

In 2010/2011 I had the privilege of being involved with three projects that aimed to explore the potential for bringing older and younger LGBT people together in 'intergenerational' work. The projects took place in Stockport (Greater Manchester), Camden (London) and Leicester, and employed distinct themes with the common aim of bringing younger and older LGBT people together in a programme of activities that would become 'multigenerational' rather than 'intergenerational'. The concept of bringing older and younger LGBT people together to enhance support and develop generational understanding was developed by Antony Smith (Age UK) who worked with colleagues based at local Age UKs, Gendered Intelligence (a group working primarily with trans young people), Leicester LGBT Centre, Stockport Youth Service, the Royal Central School of Speech and Drama, and the Universities of Salford and Leicester. An exciting aspect of being involved with these projects for all stakeholders was an understanding that this was one of the first coordinated attempts to bring younger and older LGBT people together in the UK through community-based work. Funding such a novel initiative required vision and a commitment to equality and human rights, which came in the shape of Dr Jack T. Watters (Pfizer), to whom this chapter is dedicated; this funding was matched by vInspired. With my colleague, Sally-Marie Bamford at the International Longevity Centre-UK (ILC-UK), our role was to evaluate the projects taking place.

Existing evidence of a need for strengthening intergenerational relations

One of the first activities we undertook was to examine the evidence base and establish: (1) why an intergenerational approach was needed; and (2) whether a similar approach had been adopted elsewhere. At the time (2010) we found patchy evidence (mainly US-based and using qualitative approaches) suggesting that both younger and older LGB people faced challenges compared to non-LGBT peers that could impact upon their health outcomes.

The evidence suggested that LGBT young people may not receive the same levels of support that non-LGBT people do during the transition to adulthood. For example, US data found that non-heterosexual young people receive less parental support during the (chronological) period of transitioning to adulthood than their heterosexual peers do (Needham and Austin, 2010). This lower level of parental support is also found to explain health disparities occurring early on in life such as increased risks of depressive symptomology and substance abuse (Needham and Austin, 2010). Other social relationships may also be vulnerable to strain, and LGB people experience substantially higher levels of bullying than non-LGB people as well as lower levels of life satisfaction during teenage years (Henderson, 2015).

In later adulthood, these unequal starts may continue through into different ageing 'processes' among LGBT people (e.g. Harrison, 2006), and may also help explain why and how LGB people enter into older ages with different levels of 'capital'. LGB people are more likely at age 50 to be single and to have experienced multiple cohabiting relationships of shorter duration than are non-LGBT people, a likely reflection of inadequate support services and societal hostility towards same-sex relationships over the life course (Meyer, 2003; Kneale et al., 2014). Meanwhile older LGB people have been characterised as societally invisible, and consequently underserved by formal systems of support (Fredriksen-Goldsen and Muraco, 2010). Strained relationships with non-LGBT peers, manifested through discrimination and stigma, and a perceived need for privacy and avoidance of self-disclosure, may place older LGBT people (e.g. Wilkens, 2015) and younger LGBT people (e.g. DeLonga et al., 2011) at increased risk of loneliness and social isolation. Although it is important to acknowledge the diversity in outcomes and circumstances among LGBT people (Muraco and Fredriksen-Goldsen, 2016), the evidence depicted older and younger LGBT people as navigating challenging transitions and social relationships, and both generations were likely to be facing degrees of homophobia, biphobia and transphobia in age-related settings (social care environments and schools respectively) (Potter et al., 2011). However, through its absence, UK evidence was equivocal on the state of *intergenerational* relationships among LGBT people, and their role as a mechanism in offsetting low well-being.

Similarly, the sparse evidence concerning the effectiveness of intergenerational activities and interventions was not focused on LGBT people (Potter et al., 2011). Some of the hypothesised impacts of intergenerational practice on LGBT and other groups included increased social contact, facilitation of human capital transfer, development of life skills, and the creation of culture and exchange of history (Potter et al., 2011); proponents have also emphasised the benefits of intergenerational practice for well-being (Kaplan et al., 2006; Newman and Hatton-Yeo, 2008). Routes to an improved mental well-being among intergenerational projects, applicable to older and younger people, are multifarious and include breaking down generational stereotypes, increased confidence in navigating shared spaces, greater sense of community and feeling valued within a community; and developing increased feelings of acceptance (e.g. MacCallum et al., 2010; Alcock et al., 2011; Varvarigou et al., 2011). These projects often include working towards a common goal as an element, which in itself can enable participants to develop new skills, motivations, and a new appreciation of their current knowledge and experience, which can reinforce feelings of well-being (MacCallum et al., 2010; Alcock et al., 2011; Varvarigou et al., 2011). Although there was no reason to suspect that these associations would not be generalisable to LGBT people, they remained largely untested at the time.

A disjointed evidence base suggested that LGBT social networks were structured differently, and that younger and older LGBT people faced challenges that could impact upon their well-being; however, this was largely unexplored in UK settings, particularly through quantitative methods, and evidence for transgender people was particularly scarce. Meanwhile community-level intergenerational projects had been theorised to improve younger and older participants' well-being, but were untested among LGBT people in the UK. The interventions took place despite an uncertain evidence base (see Kneale et al. (2011) for an overview), but the remainder of this chapter explores whether and how this gap in knowledge has been plugged.

New opportunities for establishing evidence of need for intergenerational work among LGBT people in the UK?

Since 2010/2011, a number of studies have started to collect data on same-sex identity and behaviour, which could allow for establishing whether a need for intergenerational work among LGBT people exists. Collection started through being able to identify same-sex cohabiting couples in large datasets (e.g. Kneale et al., 2014) and the census, although this was restricted, with partnership being a prerequisite for identification. Since then, data collection has progressed to examining sexual identity in large household studies such as the Integrated Household Survey (Joloza et al., 2010) and the UK Household Longitudinal Study (Uhrig, 2015), as well as studies focused on young people such as the Next Steps study (Henderson, 2015); or older people such as the English Longitudinal Study of Ageing (ELSA; the focus of this study) (Kneale, 2016). Many of these sources are yet to progress to examine gender identity alongside sexual identity, impeding the ability to undertake trans-inclusive research.

Using newly available data collected from people aged 50 and over in ELSA, the relationships and well-being of older people are examined for indicative evidence of a need for projects with an intergenerational focus. To gain a fuller picture of a need for intergenerational projects, corresponding analysis of a younger dataset is required, although this falls out of the remit of the present chapter. ELSA is a longitudinal study of people aged 50 and over and is the prime source of quantitative insights into the ageing process in the UK. ELSA was one of the first studies to measure older people's lifetime same-sex experiences and desires (Steptoe et al., 2013). The study originally recruited around 12,000 respondents in 2002; and in 2012 it included data on sexual experiences from a total of 6,201 respondents, for whom separate weights were constructed to account for non-response to questions on sexual attraction. ELSA is a multipurpose study and does not collect direct indicators of need and unmet need around intergenerational relations. However, we are able to assemble indicative evidence beginning with examining whether, compared to non-LGB people, LGB people aged 50-plus have similar social networks and whether they feel isolated from those around them. The analyses did not explore patterns among older transgender people due to limitations in the data, and a number of other caveats surround the findings which are discussed in full below. Many of those in these analyses would not be conventionally regarded as 'older', although a broad definition of older as including those aged 50 and over matches the criteria imposed in the intergenerational projects described earlier (Kneale et al., 2011).

Identifying older LGB people and measuring relationships

Due to a small sample size and difficulties in distinguishing behaviour taking place at different life course stages, in this chapter differences are examined between 'heterosexual' respondents (referred to as non-LGB from this point onward) and a combined category that includes 'lesbian, gay and bisexual' respondents (referred to as LGB from this point onward (see Kneale (2016) for further notes on derivation)). These categories are derived based on reports of same-sex desires and experiences. As well as overlooking transgender people, this approach means that important differences within the LGB spectrum are glossed over; however, the small sample of LGB older people precludes further exploration. The working sample size is composed of 237 people identified as LGB and 4,586 identified as non-LGB (254 and 4,933 respectively for analyses of loneliness).

To examine how older LGB people's relationships may differ from those of non-LGB people, the analysis employs a measure of exclusion from relationships originally developed by Barnes and colleagues (2006). This involves creating a score reflecting whether people reported close relationships with their partner, children, friends and other family members, as well as how often they were able to sustain this relationship with visits or phone calls (see (Barnes et al. (2006) for full details of the scoring method). A cut-off point was imposed that roughly approximated to one in ten people being denoted as excluded from social relationships. The results clearly show that those we identify as LGB are at a substantially higher risk of exclusion from social relationships than others; approximately twice as likely (7.2 per cent among non-LGB compared to 15.0 per cent among LGB older people; see Figure 8.1).

It is perhaps unsurprising, due to divergent life course trajectories (Hammack and Cohler, 2011), that Figure 8.1 shows that older LGB people are less likely to have children, a key intergenerational relationship for many older people. However, an unanticipated finding is among those with children, where there is a (non-statistically significant) trend towards lower quality relationships among LGB people compared to non-LGB people. Non-LGB people are also more likely to have grandchildren, but among those with grandchildren there are also (non-statistically significant) indications that levels of frequent contact are lower, with older LGB people less likely to have looked after their grandchildren. Table 8.1 presents odds ratios showing the likelihood of these outcomes once we account for known differences in background characteristics (age, gender

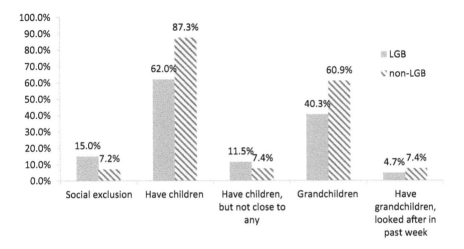

Figure 8.1 Relationship between older LGB and non-LGB people.

Sample numbers: Social exclusion, Have children; Have grandchildren (non-LGB=4584; LGB n=237); Have children, not close to any (non-LGB=4024; LGB n=153); Have grandchildren, looked after in past week (non-LGB=3074; LGB n=107); percentages are weighted.

and relationship status), which may also influence the composition and maintenance of social relationships (Cronin and King, 2010). LGB people remain significantly more likely to experience exclusion from social relationships (model 1) and not to have children and grandchildren (models 3 and 5).

Finally, the data allow for consideration of the impact that having lower density relationships may exert upon the extent to which older people report often feeling lonely: descriptively, the data suggest that older LGB people are more likely to report often feeling lonely (12.7 per cent compared to 7.0 per cent of non-LGB people). Model 6 (Table 8.1) shows that the odds of older LGB reporting often feeling lonely are over 1.7 times higher than for non-LGB people.

These findings begin to present a case for the need for projects that seek to foster social relationships among older LGB people. However, the analyses also attempt to impose a heteronormative framework for measuring the density and intensity of social relationships – a framework that does not reflect the original motivations for undertaking the intergenerational projects. Some indicators, such as feelings of loneliness, are likely to be salient universally, although the depth of indicators collected around family, partners and children collected in ELSA holds less relevance to LGB lives due

Table 8.1 Odds of experiencing different relationship statuses among older LGB and non-LGB people.

	Model 1: Odds of being excluded from social relationships	Model 2: Odds of having children	Model 3: Odds of being close to child (conditional on having a child)	Model 4: Odds of having grandchildren	Model 5: Odds of looking after grandchildren weekly (conditional on having a grandchild)	Model 6: Odds of often feeling lonely
Reference: Non-LGB	1	1	1	1	1	1
LGB	1.784*	0.270***	0.738	0.478***	0.532	1.711*
	[1.104,2.884]	[0.189,0.386]	[0.367,1.484]	[0.336,0.681]	[0.224,1.263]	[1.003,2.917]
N	4863	4863	3970	4863	3181	5829

Notes
Exponentiated coefficients; 95% confidence intervals in brackets.
* $p < 0.05$, ** $p < 0.01$, *** $p < 0.001$.
Estimates are weighted and standard errors adjusted for sample design. All models contain the following c variates: gender, relationship status, age group, employment status, household income quintile and self-rat health.

to known differences in patterns of partnership and family/social networks (Westwood, 2013; Kneale et al., 2014). New opportunities for identification of LGB (but not always 'T') people in large surveys are clearly welcome, but become of limited value for exploring LGB biographies of ageing where there is insufficient statistical power to explore intersectionalities, where significant groups remain invisible, and where the indicators themselves are not salient to LGBT life course patterns. Such indicators may themselves need 'queering' in order to become applicable to older LGB lives (Cronin and King, 2014). Therefore, while new quantitative data may hold potential to explore disparities between LGB and non-LGB people, they may not always be suitable for (queer) theory-driven enquiry that provides evidence of need.

Providing a blueprint for future intergenerational projects? A scoping review

We may now be in a better position to establish the effectiveness of taking an intergenerational approach among LGBT people, and the extent to which the evidence base has developed since 2010 is investigated here through a scoping review of the literature. The interest here is the extent to which the projects described at the beginning of this chapter represented 'early adopters' of intergenerational practice among LGBT people in the UK, or remain pioneering examples.

Two databases (Scopus[1] and ProQuest Social Sciences[2]) were searched systematically by the author in October 2017 for literature published in 2010 onward.[3] Included studies reported on community-based projects taking place in the UK among LGBT people and must have comprised an inter-generational component among both generations of LGB older and younger people (which excluded most family-based interventions and interventions around LGBT parenthood). Included were intervention studies aimed at changing or enhancing intergenerational relations, rather than observa-tional studies. The focus here was therefore exclusively on studies providing evidence of effectiveness or feasibility of LGBT intergenerational projects in the UK. Items were screened on the basis of title and abstract, and papers retrieved for studies that met the inclusion criteria, before being screened again on the basis of full text. In total, 2,111 items were screened on title and abstract, and 2,077 were excluded; this left 34 studies for which full texts were retrieved.[4] Of these 34 studies, just one study met the inclusion criteria outlined above after reading the full text (Farrier, 2015).

Evidence from similar approaches and 'near-misses'

Farrier's (2015) study reports on the understanding of temporality and the need to challenge default heteronormativity in the treatment of 'generations' through intergenerational work with LGBT people. His study provides a de-tailed account of the 'Front Room', an intergenerational performance pro-ject organised by the Royal Central School of Speech and Drama, which also developed one of the intergenerational projects presented earlier (and discussed in Chapter 9, this volume). 'Front Room' involved younger (18–25 years) and older (50–85 years) LGBT people sharing their stories; these were recorded and younger participants worked with a creative team to generate further content for a play (also supplemented by further research) which toured London and Birmingham. An explicit theme of 'Front Room' was to challenge heteronormativity around concepts of generations and inter-generational, notions of heritability and legacy, and of the way time itself shapes LGBT lives, through recognising 'queer time'. Farrier emphasised the notion of 'temporal drag' as a theoretical underpinning used to frame the way in which queer identity 'might effect change, articulate agency, and re-site itself though temporal shift' (Farrier, 2015, p. 1402). This allowed participants to disregard notions of the past as being passed but to recon-ceptualise historical events as part of current temporality and to avoid re-strictive generational metaphors. Results, in the form of empirical outcome data (quantitative or qualitative), are absent, but the study provides a discus-sion of potential theoretical underpinnings of intergenerational work with LGBT people, and the importance of re-orientating intergenerational work positively from the outset. Farrier is critical of the treatment of the 'gener-ational' in previous LGB intergenerational work (citing Potter et al., 2011; Bamford et al., 2011) in implying that generations were closed entities, the attempted establishment of 'need', and the perceived ascription of 'victim-hood' status, rather than intergenerational projects representing a greater symbolism of radicalism, unity and celebration (Farrier, 2015). His study concludes by reinforcing the utility of the use of performance art/theatre in providing a creative space for the treatment of temporality across diverse ages and identities.

Farrier's study was the only report of community-based intergenerational work taking place among LGBT people in the UK since 2010/2011, although the evidence base has developed beyond the UK. Theatre was used to unify LGB generations through examining the different stereotypes that existed in the 'Bridging the Gap' project that took place in New York (Houseal et al., 2013). Written as a case study around the dramatic strategy used (Roll on the Wall), Houseal and colleagues (2013) conclude that the method is a 'powerful, multifaceted tool, well suited to our intergenerational LGBTQ participants' (Houseal et al., 2013, p. 207). In another US example, participants of an inter-generational long-term 'literature discussion group' (book group) discussed various LGBT texts (Blackburn and Clark, 2011). Other interventions taking place elsewhere included befriending and mentoring programmes (Rummell, 2013; Gilles, 2011) and a psychological/counselling intervention (Friedman, 2014), each incorporating an intergenerational dimension.

One notable addition was the 'It Gets Better' project, the online support project providing young LGBT people with support from adults, which started in response to a string of suicides among (US) LGBT youth. Given its online nature, its impact has been felt in the UK and more localised initi-atives have since developed modelled on 'It Gets Better'.[5] A number of stud-ies have examined the impact of 'It Gets Better' (Phillips, 2013; Hurley, 2014; Jones, 2015). While the initiative is intended to support LGBT youth, one study examined the impact upon video makers themselves, revealing collat-eral benefits among video makers, including increased feelings of generativ-ity and feelings of empowerment in being able to contact and discuss LGBT issues with younger people (Hurley, 2014). However, some authors have also been critical of the content of 'It Gets Better' videos in masking intersec-tionalities of race, class, gender and sexual identity, the exclusion of which may actually serve to perpetuate feelings of isolation among some LGBT young people (Phillips, 2013). Goltz's (2013) critical examination of 'It Gets Better' questions the extent to which a discursive focus on breaking the link between LGBT youth and suicide actually serves to reify the association. Nonetheless, he also concludes that the project offers a 'tapestry of experi-ences that testify to multiple forms of family, friendship, community, and support systems that may seem currently unimaginable to isolated queer youths' (Goltz, 2013, p. 143). The evidence remains sparse on the impact of 'It Gets Better' upon the well-being of young LGBT people themselves.

Finally, in addition to the literature around the effectiveness and feasibil-ity of intergenerational work, evidence that could be used to provide a case for intergenerational work is burgeoning in the UK. Much of this evidence provides an insight into challenges faced by younger and older LGBT people that may also incorporate a 'generational' component. Among older people, these have included studies on the complexity of LGBT social networks and the challenge that older LGBT people may have when negotiating legal structures and services due to the complexity of these networks (Westwood, 2013, 2015); studies that have examined methods of knowledge exchange between older people and service providers (King, 2015); as well as a number of studies focussed on aspects of care and caring relationships (Cronin et al., 2011; King and Cronin, 2013; Parslow and Hegarty, 2013; Tinker et al., 2014). Some studies also reinforce the complexity of thinking about LGBT in terms of 'generations' and reinforce calls for challenging mainstream concepts in ageing literature (Cronin and King, 2010); for example, Hughes and Deutsch's (2010) study on 'older' gay men's holiday preferences included men aged 35 years and over, undermining approaches that conceptualise younger and older as closed and distinct groups.[6] However, there remain a number of evidence gaps, particularly around younger and older transgender people's life course trajectories.

Reflections on the evidence base for further intergenerational work among LGBT people

In the context of the current chapter, presenting a need for greater intergenerational work and demonstrating the effectiveness of interventions can secure funding for further research and interventions, projects and services that facilitate contact between generations. For intergenerational projects, this may involve working to influence decision makers at different tiers of government as well as across areas of policy that have traditionally operated in silo. This makes having robust evidence all the more important for intergenerational projects. Local government bodies, which may be the very agencies to fund future intergenerational work and LGBT services, have experienced cuts in funding of around 40 per cent since 2011/2012 (Local Government Association, 2014) in a period of prolonged austerity. In such a climate, decision makers will increasingly be seeking evidence of need, effectiveness and cost-effectiveness, and may be seeking higher thresholds of evidence before committing funding for services commissioned (see also Chapters 12 and 13, this volume).

For those advocating further intergenerational work, there is a mismatch between the evidence base and the type of evidence that may influence decision making. Since 2010/2011 there has been a greatly expanded literature exploring generational challenges among LGBT people. Progress has also been made in enhancing the availability of data that allows the exploration of LGB lives in quantitative studies, which has been utilised by some (Uhrig, 2015) and may help illuminate evidence of need for LGB-targeted initiatives. The example provided here using data from ELSA illuminated disparities in feelings of loneliness between LGB and non-LGB people, which in turn could theoretically be offset through strengthening intergenerational relations and solidarity. However, there exist common limitations to the scope of analyses possible in such data, based around sample size, the visibility of transgender people and the salience of the indicators available.

In contrast, we have seen only limited development in the evidence base measuring the impact of intergenerational work among LGBT people in the UK, with a particular failure in addressing questions of effectiveness. Effectiveness in this sense need not necessarily reflect hard outcomes measured quantitatively, but can also reflect feelings of satisfaction and change as a result of participation in intergenerational work or the reach of projects across different intersectionalities (Kneale et al., 2011). Published studies have omitted to include information on outputs or outcomes that occur as a result of participation, and may have actively avoided measuring change and outcomes of participation, as this could imply a need for change, which in turn may contribute to a 'victim trope'. This is not to say that the evidence base has not changed in important ways through the expansion of theoretical frameworks that can underpin LGBT intergenerational projects (e.g. Farrier, 2015), as well as the development of tools that can facilitate the process (Houseal et al., 2013). It nevertheless remains questionable the extent to which such evidence meets the needs of decision makers and funders, as opposed to aiding practitioners who are already invested in the idea of working intergenerationally with LGBT people. Clearly the needs of both groups of stakeholders must be met if we are to secure funding for future work and services and to improve the quality of these experiences.

There are limitations to the above findings. In the quantitative analyses it was not possible to explore differences within the LGB spectrum, to identify transgender individuals, and the analysis undertaken was a complete case analysis. In terms of the scoping review, the caveats to the results include the possibility that the searches were conducted on too narrow a body of literature; that the results were screened by a single reviewer; and that intergenerational LGBT studies may have been conducted in the UK but that the evidence may not be published.

Conclusion

The exploration of quantitative data collected from older people presented here (albeit based on one source with caveats) was highly suggestive of a need for interventions that aid brokering social relationships among older LGBT people to offset disproportionately high levels of loneliness. The collection of indicators salient to LGBT life course research could further the potential utility of these sources. These analyses also took place in the context of an expanded body of evidence that illuminates generational challenges. However, current policy towards austerity means that projects and services have to demonstrate both a need for intergenerational work among LGBT people *and* its benefits.

Intergenerational practice among LGBT people is likely to be an important vehicle for improving the life chances of younger people as well as reducing inequalities and emerging social challenges among older people. Qualitative findings uncovered in the evaluation of the three pioneering intergenerational projects demonstrate the power of this model in providing mutual support and vehicles for creative expression, celebrating shared history and differences in identity, and promoting feelings of intergenerational trust, and, for some, individual well-being; they also demonstrate that an intergenerational approach is fun, feasible and, ultimately, fundable (Kneale et al., 2011). In the absence of further developments in the evidence base, these projects remain relatively isolated examples of the potential capacity of intergenerational projects to change the outcomes of both younger and older LGBT people.

While 'evidence' as we know it is not the sole determinant of decision making, there may be more that we can do as generators of evidence to bridge this gap. Ultimately the findings and arguments in this chapter support 'queering' the collection of data on LGBT people to ensure that quantitative indicators reflect LGBT experiences, as well as 'policing' the way in which intervention findings are reported. The latter is particularly important to ensure that in addition to contributing to important theoretical debates within LGBT literature, the results of intergenerational work reach wider audiences and have currency with a broader set of stakeholders.

Notes

1 http://www.scopus.com/.
2 http://search.proquest.com/socialsciences/subjects/advanced.
3 Search strings available on request.
4 One code was selected per item but items could fall into multiple categories.
5 See LGBT Youth Scotland Video Series: www.lgbtyouth.org.uk/m-yp-it-gets-better.
6 Similar studies were also uncovered in Potter et al. (2011).

References

Alcock, CL., Camic, PM., Barker, C. et al. (2011) 'Intergenerational practice in the community: A focused ethnographic evaluation', *Journal of Community & Applied Social Psychology,* 21(5): 419–432.

Bamford, S-M., Kneale, D. and Diener, L. (2011) *Intergenerational Projects for the LGBT Community: A Toolkit for Practice.* London: International Longevity Centre UK.

Barnes, M., Blom, A., Cox, K. et al. (2006) *The Social Exclusion of Older People: Evidence from the First Wave of the English Longitudinal Study of Ageing (ELSA): Final Report.* London: Office of the Deputy Prime Minister.

Blackburn, MV. and Clark, CT. (2011) 'Analyzing Talk in a long-term literature discussion group: Ways of operating within LGBT-inclusive and queer discourses', *Reading Research Quarterly,* 46(3): 222–248.

Cronin, A. and King, A. (2010) 'Power, inequality and identification: Exploring diversity and intersectionality amongst older LGB adults', *Sociology*, 44(5): 876–892.

Cronin, A. and King, A. (2014) 'Only connect? Older lesbian, gay and bisexual (LGB) adults and social capital', *Ageing and Society*, 34(2): 258–279.

Cronin, A., Ward, R., Pugh, S. et al. (2011) 'Categories and their consequences: Understanding and supporting the caring relationships of older lesbian, gay and bisexual people', *International Social Work*, 54(3): 421–435.

DeLonga, K., Torres, HL., Kamen, C. et al. (2011) 'Loneliness, internalized homophobia, and compulsive internet use: Factors associated with sexual risk behavior among a sample of adolescent males seeking services at a community LGBT center', *Sexual Addiction & Compulsivity*, 18(2): 61–74.

Farrier, S. (2015) 'Playing with time: Gay intergenerational performance work and the productive possibilities of queer temporalities', *Journal of Homosexuality*, 62(10): 1398–1418.

Fredriksen-Goldsen, KI. and Muraco, A. (2010) 'Aging and sexual orientation: A 25-year review of the literature', *Research on Aging*, 32(3): 372–413.

Friedman, RJ. (2014) 'A phenomenological study of a psychoeducational workshop for gay men: Participating in the Father Hunger Workshop'. Pacifica Graduate Institute.

Gilles, JM. (2011) *A theoretical rationale for the development of a mentoring relationship between PFLAG parents and LGBQ adolescents and emerging adults with family-of-origin conflict or rejection*. Spalding University.

Goltz, DB. (2013) 'It gets better: Queer futures, critical frustrations, and radical potentials', *Critical Studies in Media Communication*, 30(2): 135–151.

Hammack, PL. and Cohler, BJ. (2011) 'Narrative, identity, and the politics of exclusion: Social change and the gay and lesbian life course', *Sexuality Research and Social Policy*, 8: 162–182.

Harrison, J. (2006) 'Coming out ready or not! Gay, lesbian, bisexual, transgender and intersex ageing and aged care in Australia: Reflections, contemporary developments and the road ahead', *Gay and Lesbian Issues and Psychology Review*, 2: 44–53.

Henderson, M. (2015) Understanding Bullying Experiences among Sexual Minority Youths in England. London: Centre for Longitudinal Studies.

Houseal, J., Ray, K. and Teitelbaum, S. (2013) 'Identifying, confronting and disrupting stereotypes: Role on the Wall in an intergenerational LGBTQ applied theatre project', *Research in Drama Education: The Journal of Applied Theatre and Performance*, 18(2): 204–208.

Hughes, HL. and Deutsch, R. (2010) 'Holidays of older gay men: Age or sexual orientation as decisive factors?', *Tourism Management*, 31(4): 454–463.

Hughes, M. and Kentlyn, S. (2011) 'Older LGBT people's care networks and communities of practice: A brief note', *International Social Work*, 54(3): 436–444.

Hurley, SJ. (2014) 'Public pedagogy and the experience of video creators in the It Gets Better Project', *ProQuest Dissertations and Theses*, Ann Arbor, 222.

Izuhara, M. (2010) *Ageing and Intergenerational Relations: Family Reciprocity from a Global Perspective*. Bristol: Policy Press.

Joloza, T., Evans, J., O'Brien, R. et al. (2010) *Measuring Sexual Identity: An Evaluation Report*. Newport: Office for National Statistics.

Jones, RH. (2015) 'Generic intertextuality in online social activism: The case of the It Gets Better project', *Language in Society*, 44(3): 317–339.

Kaplan, M. (1997) 'The benefits of intergenerational community service projects: Implications for promoting intergenerational unity, community activism, and cultural continuity', *Journal of Gerontological Social Work,* 28(3): 211–228.

Kaplan, M., Liu, S-T. and Hannon, P. (2006) 'Intergenerational engagement in retirement communities: A case study of a community capacity-building model', *Journal of Applied Gerontology,* 25(5): 406–426.

King, A. (2015) 'Prepare for impact? Reflecting on knowledge exchange work to improve services for older LGBT people in times of austerity', *Social Policy and Society,* 14(1): 15–27.

King, A. and Cronin, A. (2013) 'Queering care in later life: The lived experiences and intimacies of older lesbian, gay and bisexual adults', in Sanger, T. and Taylor, Y. (eds), *Mapping Intimacies: Relations, Exchanges, Affects.* Basingstoke: Palgrave Macmillan, pp. 112–129.

Kneale, D. (2016) 'Connected communities? LGB older people and their risk of exclusion from decent housing and neighbourhoods', *Quality in Ageing and Older Adults,* 17(2): 107–118.

Kneale, D., Serra, V., Bamford, S-M. et al. (2011) *Celebrating Intergenerational Diversity.* London: International Longevity Centre-UK.

Kneale, D., Sholl, P., Sherwood, C. et al. (2014) 'Ageing and lesbian, gay and bisexual relationships', *Working with Older People,* 18(3): 142–151.

Local Government Association. (2014) *Under Pressure: How Councils are Planning for Future Cuts.* London: Local Government Association.

MacCallum, J., Palmer, D., Wright, P. et al. (2010) 'Australian perspectives: Community building through intergenerational exchange programs', *Journal of Intergenerational Relationships,* 8(2): 113–127.

Meyer, IH. (2003) 'Prejudice, social stress, and mental health in lesbian, gay, and bisexual populations: Conceptual issues and research evidence', *Psychological Bulletin,* 129(5): 674.

Muraco, A. and Fredriksen-Goldsen, KI. (2016) 'Turning points in the lives of lesbian and gay adults age 50 and over', *Advances in Life Course Research,* 30:124–132.

Needham, BL. and Austin, EL. (2010) 'Sexual orientation, parental support, and health during the transition to young adulthood', *Journal of Youth and Adolescence,* 39(10): 1189–1198.

Newman, S. and Hatton-Yeo, A. (2008) 'Intergenerational learning and the contributions of older people', *Ageing Horizons,* 8: 31–39.

Parslow, O. and Hegarty, P. (2013) 'Who cares? UK lesbian caregivers in a heterosexual world', *Women's Studies International Forum,* 40: 78–86.

Phillips, LM. (2013) *A multi-method Examination of Race, Class, Gender, Sexual Orientation, and Motivations for Participation in the YouTube-based 'It Gets Better Project'.* ProQuest Dissertations and Theses, Ann Arbor, 281.

Potter, C., Bamford, S. and Kneale, D. (2011) *Bridging the Gap: Exploring the Potential for Bringing Older and Younger LGBT People Together.* London: International Longevity Centre.

Reczek, C. (2014) 'The intergenerational relationships of gay men and lesbian women', *The Journals of Gerontology Series B: Psychological Sciences and Social Sciences,* 69(6): 909–919.

Rummell, CL. (2013) *A Unique Support for Sexual-minority Identity Development: An Interpretative Phenomenological Analysis of a Long-term Formal Mentoring*

Relationship Between an Adult and a Youth From the Gay Community. Portland State University.

Simpson, P. (2013) 'Alienation, ambivalence, agency: Middle-aged gay men and ageism in Manchester's gay village', *Sexualities*, 16(3–4): 283–299.

Steptoe, A., Breeze, E., Banks, J. et al. (2013) 'Cohort profile: The English longitudinal study of ageing', *International Journal of Epidemiology*, 42(6): 1640–1648.

Tinker, A., Gilani, N., Luthra, I. et al. (2014) 'Why is it important to consider so-called "invisible" older people in UK healthcare?', *Quality in Ageing and Older Adults*, 15(4): 187–196.

Uhrig, S. (2015) 'Sexual orientation and poverty in the UK: A review and top-line findings from the UK household longitudinal study', *Journal of Research Gender Studies*, 5(1): 23–72.

Varvarigou, M., Creech, A., Hallam, S. et al. (2011) 'Bringing different generations together in music-making: An intergenerational music project in East London', *International Journal of Community Music*, 4(3): 207–220.

Westwood, S. (2013) '"My friends are my family": An argument about the limitations of contemporary law's recognition of relationships in later life', *Journal of Social Welfare and Family Law*, 35: 347–363.

Westwood, S. (2015) 'Complicating kinship and inheritance: Older lesbians' and gay men's Will-writing in England', *Feminist Legal Studies*, 23: 181–197.

Wilkens, J. (2015) 'Loneliness and belongingness in older lesbians: The role of social groups as "community"', *Journal of Lesbian Studies*, 19: 90–101.

9 A complex matrix of identities

Working intergenerationally with LGBTQ people

Catherine McNamara

Introduction

Intergenerational project work is an established field, and often involves the arts as a medium for exploration and articulation of particular lived experiences (Epstein and Boisvert, 2001; Hatton-Yeo, 2006; Lloyd, 2008; Springate et al., 2008). In this chapter, I will draw upon a number of examples of intergenerational practice and research that have influenced my own work in this area. The chapter takes the *INTERarts project* as a key example. This was an intergenerational project that I co-facilitated in 2010 to 2011 as part of a collaboration between The Royal Central School of Speech and Drama (University of London) and Gendered Intelligence.

Gendered Intelligence (GI) formally registered as a Community Interest Company (CIC) in 2008. A CIC is a specific type of company structure in the UK which reinvests profits in the company for community and social benefit rather than for shareholders. Dr Jay Stewart and I were co-founders and Stewart is the Chief Executive Officer (CEO) for the organisation. The aims of GI are to increase the quality of young trans people's lives and to raise awareness of their needs across the UK and beyond. In working towards those aims, we seek to contribute to the creation of community cohesion and strength across the whole of the trans community throughout the UK, and to generate discussion and debate around gender, inequality rooted in gender, misogyny, misandry and sexism. Our position is that gender is a construct and not a natural phenomenon. It is a system which presents challenges in everyday life for the majority of people, regardless of individuals' trans or cisgender status. Here, 'cisgender' is the adjective that relates to a person whose self-identity conforms with the gender that corresponds to their biological sex. In this chapter, 'trans' is used to mean a broad spectrum of gender identities and gendered expressions, and to include people who feel their gender identity does not sit comfortably with the sex they were assigned at birth, including, but not limited to, transgender and non-binary identified people. Not all non-binary identified people would identify as trans and, as an umbrella term, trans does not suit all people in the same way.

GI carries out arts-based programmes and creative workshops with and for young trans people and, on occasion, with young LGBQ (Lesbian, Gay, Bisexual and Queer) people from across the UK, including providing some opportunities for people over the age of 25. The intergenerational project under discussion in this chapter is one such example from 2010; others include *The Sci:dentity project*, 2006 to 2007 (Rooke, 2010); *Brief Encounters Theatre in Education project*, 2009 to 2012 (Greer, 2012); *i:trans: Constructing Selves Through Technology*, 2012; *GI's Anatomy*, 2013 (McNay and Stewart, 2015) and *Transvengers*, 2014 to 2015 (Wellcome Collection, 2015; Sandell, 2017). These projects invariably involve collaboration with partners who have included the Science Museum, the Wellcome Gallery, the Fringe Benefits Theatre Company (based in Los Angeles, USA) and London Drawing (Gendered Intelligence, 2009–2017).

Within intergenerational practice, there is a strong emphasis on differing lived experiences on the basis of age, and the idea that people from one generation or distinct age group, be that younger or older people, tend to have reduced contact with those at the opposite point of the age scale. Intergenerational work seeks to provide opportunities for both older and younger people to benefit from spending time with each other and engaging in some kind of joint activity. Lloyd (2008) argues that social contact, human capital transfers (i.e. the exchange of knowledge and skills), and the creation of culture and exchange of history are among the many outcomes linked to intergenerational practice. He states that 'intergenerational transfers and exchanges within families have long been a topic of interest to academic researchers. However, such transfers can also occur at the community and societal levels' (Lloyd, 2008, p. 2).This chapter explores the range of intentions and outcomes that have underpinned a number of community-based intergenerational projects.

The *INTERarts project* involved working intergenerationally with people who identify as lesbian, gay, bisexual, trans and/or queer (LGBTQ). Intergenerational work with LGBTQ participants is relatively unprecedented; I developed ways of thinking about the 'matrix of identities' at the centre of the *INTERarts project* as we planned the creative processes and as I reflected on the practice retrospectively. Identities in this project were intergenerational, inter-sexuality and inter-gender, and this chapter identifies the specific challenges of working with such a diversity of identities within intergenerational LGBTQ work. It offers specific indications as to how to negotiate those challenges and demonstrates the ways in which the lessons from this project might inform other work in the areas of LGBTQ arts and activism, applied theatre, community arts and intergenerational work more broadly. The chapter seeks to consolidate and critically reflect on the *INTERarts project* and share a model of practice that may be used by other practitioner-researchers in this and cognate fields.

Intergenerational arts practice

Intergenerational arts practice is wide-ranging in its aims and its specific focus. A project will often bring older and younger people from a particular cultural group together, for example, to explore a specific topic or theme such as the history of the local community. By way of an example, and to position the *INTERarts project* as an LGBTQ intergenerational project in relation to other work in this field, it is useful to draw upon a range of projects that show differing practices and specific themes. *Zekenim: Honoring and Celebrating Los Angeles' Jewish Elders* (2016) is an intergenerational art programme designed to illuminate the life stories of older Jewish people living in and around the city. This project is funded by a grant from the Jewish Community Foundation of Los Angeles to the University of Southern California, Davis School of Gerontology. As well as the culturally specific nature of the project, the model of the practice is very particular. The project seeks to bring older people together with younger artists and facilitate the telling of stories as inspiration for the artists to create a piece of art in their own medium of choice.

Sadie E. Rubin and colleagues talk about the ways in which intergenerational work can support younger participants to challenge their assumptions about ageing, reflect on their own ageing and begin to feel 'more comfortable with the idea of getting older' (Rubin et al., 2015, p. 248). Challenging gerontophobia and ageism was a more explicit intention in the Promoting Art for Life Enrichment Through Transgenerational Engagement (PALETTE) project led by Rubin than it is in other projects; nevertheless, much intergenerational work seeks to facilitate greater understanding of and between older and younger participants.

Desh is an Asian intergenerational arts project by the Asian Arts Agency based in Bristol in the UK, and has a similar model of practice to *Zekenim*. *Desh* launched at Bristol's Watershed in October 2013 and was funded by the Heritage Lottery. The term 'Desh' refers to a person's or people's native or homeland or motherland, or country (in Hindi and Urdu). This project encouraged 'Young British Asians from Bristol and the surrounding areas [to speak] with Asian elders to collect their oral histories', and to explore 'the theme of "homeland" through the creation of digital stories' (Asian Arts Agency, 2017). Young people participated in a series of skills development workshops and made films and oral history pieces based on people's memories of migration to the UK, their lives growing up in a multicultural English city in the 1980s and so forth. The work was exhibited at the city's M-shed Museum and is hosted on the Asian Arts Agency website.

Elders Share the Arts (ESTA) is a private non-profit community arts organisation based in New York City (Intergenerational Arts, 2016). The organisation runs a range of arts activities for older people, including intergenerational projects. ESTA was founded in 1979 by Susan Perlstein who went on to found the National Centre for Creative Aging (NCCA) in 2001.

History Alive (Generating Community) is an example of an intergenerational project that aimed to create cross-generational and cross-cultural connections in Brooklyn, 'using oral history as a basis for artistic expression that brings healing not only for the individual, but for society as a whole' (Perlstein and Bliss, 1994, p. 5). The project sought to engage younger and older participants in 'interdisciplinary and curriculum-based analysis that enriches their social consciousness and their capacity for creative expression' (ESTA, 2016). In a similar vein, *Frames of Brick Lane* (Magic Me, 2015)[1] brought together a group of 12 older people living in Brick Lane, East London and 12 Year 3 (ages 7 and 8) pupils from Christ Church Primary School in Brick Lane to explore the 'living history' of the area before creating a series of large-scale paintings based on their explorations. The group met weekly over the summer term to tell stories, create poetry, and draw and make maps in preparation for painting. This model facilitates all participants to be engaged in the art making as opposed to younger people using art to respond to the older people's stories. When formulating an intergenerational project design, the decisions relating to the specific model of practice, the ways in which older and young participants will engage with each other and the focus or theme of the work they will undertake are critical factors.

While many intergenerational arts projects address social cohesion in urban areas, the *Maugherow Project*, which began in 1998, was an ambitious long-term programme working in an 'expansive rural community' which engaged with cohesion of a different kind with a population of approximately 750 dispersed across a peninsula 12 miles north of Sligo town in Ireland (O Connor, 2002, p. 5). The project was initiated by the Arts Office of Sligo County Council in partnership with St Patrick's National School and supported by the North Western Health Board. The average age of older participants was 75. In the initial project phases of 1998 to 2001, the project was coordinated by Ann O Connor who is also the author of the Resource Pack associated with the project. Arts Development worker Catherine Fanning explains the aim and structure of the project:

> The project was set up in order to explore the potential of using the arts in a school environment to address the isolation and exclusion, experienced by many older people in rural areas. It was considered essential that this project would be structured in a holistic way, that would not only benefit the older people involved, but also the school, its students and the wider community.
>
> (Fanning, 2016)

One outcome of the project was the formation of Maugherow Active Age Group, an arts and activity group for older residents of Maugherow, which still meets and participates in projects. The project identified the needs of younger and older participants around teaching and nurturing, but also around communicating cultural mores and identity. In the resource pack entitled *Unwrapping Creativity: An Intergenerational approach (pilot phase 1998–2001)* (O Connor, 2002), the project team report that both older and younger generations enjoyed contact with the other age group, young and older participants experienced increased personal and creative confidence, and older people felt a decreased sense of isolation and a greater sense of well-being (100 per cent reported making new friends). The model of practice, which enabled all participants to engage in all stages of the creative activities, to make work in a new social environment and to exhibit their work for an invited audience, were elements that influenced my thinking in relation to the *INTERarts project*.

At the time the *INTERarts project* took place (2010), there were no other intergenerational projects that involved LGBTQ participants of which the project team and the external evaluation team were aware. In co-editing a themed issue of *Research in Drama Education: The Journal of Applied Theatre and Performance* in 2012, I came to learn about *Bridging the Gap*, an intergenerational LGBTQ theatre project in New York City that sought to counter the splintering of LGBTQ people into age-segregated micro-communities which deprive them 'of opportunities to weave a common history and share strategies that community members have used to survive and thrive' (Houseal et al., 2013, p.111). The project was facilitated by a team of three students from the City University of New York (CUNY) School of Professional Studies' MA in Applied Theatre programme, as a partnership between CUNY and SAGE (Services and Advocacy for Gay, Lesbian, Bisexual and Transgender Elders). The culmination of the project was a live performance of 'Step Right Up!', an original devised theatre piece presented at the Lesbian, Gay, Bisexual and Transgender Community Centre in New York City.

The *INTERarts project*

During a six-month period, from autumn 2010 to spring 2011, the three intergenerational projects, of which *INTERarts* was one, were apparently among 'the first of their kind in the UK' (Potter et al., 2011, p. 6). The projects were based in Camden (London), Stockport and Leicester. These projects aimed to promote solidarity and improve relations between different generations of the LGBTQ community. The projects were supported with funding from vInspired and Pfizer.[2] The project in Leicester used interviews conducted by younger participants to gather and record personal histories of older LGBT individuals. In Stockport, different generations of LGBT people were involved in researching and developing local policies, including raising their issues and experiences with local service providers. In Camden, we carried out the *INTERarts project*. I was Project Coordinator alongside Dr Jay Stewart and, for this project, we worked in partnership with Age UK's LGBT information and support project, Opening Doors London, which operates 'with and for older Lesbian, Gay, Bisexual and Trans people in the UK' (Opening Doors London, 2014).

All three UK projects aimed to enable older and younger people to share and learn new skills, improve understanding between younger and older LGBT people, and to foster mutual support, thereby reducing social isolation and celebrating LGBT heritage.

As Project Coordinators, we employed a small team of additional facilitators and, between us, we brought skills and experience in the areas of applied arts facilitation (inclusive and participatory practice), photography, multi-media installation art, devised performance, fine art, writing, voice, film making and film editing. As a project team, working to the aforementioned overarching project aims, we were specifically seeking to give young LGBT and queer-identified people an opportunity to further their own understanding of and pride in the heritage of their communities. Encouraging people from different generations from the LGBTQ communities to learn together by sharing stories and exploring heritage, history and culture across the decades was a new endeavour for Gendered Intelligence. The intergenerational aspect of the project gave us the opportunity to develop our own practice in new ways.

Project workshops took place over four Saturdays, culminating in an exhibition of work created by the participants. Approximately 100 people attended the exhibition, and subsequently we documented the project and this exhibition event online (Gendered Intelligence, 2013). The artworks created during the workshops that were later exhibited included live performance, installation art, photography, poster art and film. Each piece of work made was an articulation of the artist's reflections on the ways age and ageing plays a part in forming one's gender identity and sexuality. Collectively, the works offer a set of multiple perspectives on the ways that different genders and sexualities are expressed across our aged (younger and older) bodies.

Approximately 30 people participated in the project. There was an equal split between older (50-plus years) and younger (under 25) people, with participants' ages ranging from 16 to 86 years. Every participant self-identified their sexual orientation as lesbian, gay, bisexual, pan-sexual, polysexual, asexual, for example, and indeed, heterosexual. In terms of gender identity, some participants identified as transgender, as genderqueer, as non-binary, as men, as women, as gender-fluid, to give some examples. Self-identification happened across a range of levels: first, when people responded to the outreach activities and the publicity material about the project and expressed an interest in being involved, because this was being described as an LGBTQ project; second, when participants completed the project monitoring and evaluation materials and were asked questions about themselves; and third, most overtly and significantly, throughout the project sessions because gender identity and sexuality were key themes and participants were invited to reflect and comment on those themes in relation to their own lived experiences as part of a creative process.

Inclusion of all of those identity categories within a group of project participants is not straightforward, as the complexity of inclusion must take account of numerous factors within any group. In this case, the expectations people have when they begin to engage with a LGBT project – what they think it will be like and what they want from such an engagement – was a factor. Where sexual orientation and gender identity intersect in a group setting, and the group will be working in a way that foregrounds those aspects of people's identities and requires people to think and talk about them, structure can facilitate those intersections and exchanges. Structured frameworks can help individual participants engage with the project themes and with each other in more specific ways than if people are left to co-participate in creative activities in the expectation that interactions and interpersonal exchanges will come about.

Gender, sexuality, age: the paradox of the category

In specific relation to the term or category 'transgender', Henry Rubin asserts that:

> Socio-cultural categories of experience are subject to alteration as individuals try to place themselves within those categories. The newly consolidated FTM [Female-to-Male] category is already being challenged by individuals with unorthodox experiences attempting to inhabit it [...] these categories are in a perpetual dialectical motion with no final end.
>
> (Rubin, 2003, p. 142)

Inhabiting bodies and categories are the complex processes that this practice grapples with, as are some of the ways in which performance and the articulation of a subject position through the medium of art contributes to the dialectical motion of such bodies and categories. The categories of lesbian, bisexual, woman, man, gay man, trans woman, non-binary person – the categories of experience chosen and utilised by the participants in this project – are wide-ranging, fluid and certainly not fixed in their meaning.

That said, categorisation is useful to me as a researcher, because it is a constructive organising principle in everyday life, even taking account of the fluidity of identity and self-definition. Where individual people find it productive to self-identify as trans or LGBT or as 'older' in some way, for example, grouping and categorising is worthwhile in the process of coming to reflect and draw meaning from my experience as a Project Coordinator for the *INTERarts project*. To problematise the act of categorising is, however, of critical importance, and is something that numerous individuals who feature in the discussions treated in this chapter engaged in as part of their art making and their everyday lives. Categorisation is context-specific, and 'trans' as an example of a category has evolved through time and in relation to other categories. For example, David Valentine discusses the 'origin(s) and meaning(s) of transgender' in the opening chapter of *Imagining Transgender: An Ethnography of a Category*, and points to standard accounts of the history of the term in 1970s America. He also looks to academic discourse of the 1990s, socio-political activism and to shifts later in the 1990s around the use of the collective sense of the category and the lived experiences it attempts to contain and describe as 'part of organisational schema' (Valentine, 2007, p. 34). Valentine also acknowledges that transgender exists in relation to (and often to some degree in opposition to), other newer categories, such as 'genderqueer' (p. 254). *Genderqueer* is an alternative term that gained currency through the early 2000s and describes someone who identifies as a gender other than 'man' or 'woman', or someone who identifies as neither, both or some combination thereof. In relation to the man/woman binary, people identifying as genderqueer generally identify as more 'both/and' or 'neither/nor', rather than 'either/or' man or woman. As with other historically derogative terms of abuse, *queer* has not been and is not universally accepted as a positive term and is rejected by some individuals as still being injurious and offensive, and the connection to past usage of this word is inescapable: 'when the injurious term injures (and let me be clear that I think it does), it works its injury precisely through the accumulation and dissimulation of its force' (Butler, 1997, p. 52).

Valentine was writing in 2007 and since then more categories have been produced. At the moment of writing (January 2016) Facebook UK offers upward of 71 different options to describe gender identity in a user profile (Williams, 2014). 'Non-binary' is an identity category used increasingly to describe a gender identity which resists the notion that gender consists of just two binary opposites, male and female. I am consciously utilising identity categories in this chapter in order to make use of the fact that categories can create meaning, while at the same time using categories in the ways that participants used them: critically and to test the borders of their meanings and the multiple ways they can be understood, applied, refuted and challenged. Susan Stryker and Stephen Whittle (2006, p. 3) write about the term *transgender*, for example, as a term of choice for:

> a wide range of phenomena that call attention to the fact that 'gender', as it is lived, embodied, experienced, performed, and encountered, is more complex and varied than can be accounted for by the currently dominant binary sex/gender ideology of Eurocentric modernity.

A key aim of the *INTERarts project* also connected with the idea of the micro-communities within what may be thought of as a bigger, broader LGBT community. The aim was to improve understanding and relationships between younger and older LGBTQ people. 'LGBTQ' as an acronym tends to have a homogenising effect on a group of individuals who are thus described. Using people's own descriptions of themselves taken from the project monitoring forms: the participants in this project included Michelle, a 61-year-old trans woman; Val, a 70-year-old lesbian; Syriah who was 22 and stated that they did not specify their gender or sexual orientation, using 'Trans Advocate and Gender Enthusiast' to offer some form of description of themselves; Isaac was a 20-year-old trans man whose sexual orientation he described as queer; Emma was 16 and gay; Liam was a 24-year-old asexual/queer transguy; Vince was 51 and bisexual, and Sofia was 22 and a lesbian. The multiplicity within the LGBTQ acronym and specifically within this group of participants in an intergenerational LGBTQ project can be fully appreciated from this list.

Intergenerational, inter-sexuality, inter-gender arts practice

During the planning for the *INTERarts project*, a member of the *Opening Doors Camden* team talked about the older men's group and the older women's group, telling us that these two groups were not in the habit of mixing. We were advised by the project worker that we should plan men-only sessions and women-only sessions within our project to accommodate what was described as the preferences of the group members. This notion of working in discrete groups was at odds with the fundamental approach we had planned to adopt with this project, which was to bring people with different lived experiences together to work collaboratively. We acknowledged that there are numerous benefits when working in clearly defined groups, whether this was a trans youth group, a women-only space or a project for any specific marginalised group. In fact, we often work in this way. However, through this project the intention was to create a structured opportunity to work in a manner that facilitated people's exchanges with others. Moreover, it was intended that those exchanges with people whose lived experience is markedly different from one's own in terms of gender as well as age and sexual orientation were intended to be positive, enjoyable exchanges that would stimulate creative work and bring new insights into another person's subject position. We took the advice of the project worker into account and made a point of being very clear about this approach when we visited the groups as part of the outreach phase of the project. We were conscious that not everybody would be interested in working in mixed groups, but by explaining the benefits as we saw them, we were seeking to be transparent while people were forming their expectations of the project. Towards the end of project after having attended all five days, one older lesbian woman said:

> I was quite pleased really because I usually only choose to socialise with women and lesbians. So I was quite pleased that I was doing this because I was just stretching myself a bit. I found it okay, because it's not in your face because you're both focussing on something you do and it's not turned into a big thing or anything.

> (Kneale et al., 2011, p. 26)

On the subject of working alongside an older person, a younger participant reflected on the experience of working alongside the older lesbians, gay men, bisexual and trans people:

> I think I am more positive about growing older because I am seeing more people in the older LGBTQ community and I am realising that you don't get old and decrepit and die [...] you become quite beautiful and you evolve as a person.
>
> (Kneale at al., 2011, p.58)

To provide a greater insight into this process of developing one person's understanding of another person and cultivating one's relationship with someone with a different set of experiences, I am going to talk about Elizabeth and Isaac. Elizabeth was an older lesbian who is cisgender (a person whose self-identity conforms with the gender that corresponds to their biological sex), and Isaac was a younger trans man who identified as queer. They expressed very different lived experiences, not only in the length of time they have lived (their respective ages), but also their sexual orientations and their gender identities. Working together through the *INTERarts project*, they made the short film *Queer Voices* (Clarke and Gustafsson Wood, 2011). The film explores gender identity, sexuality and age through voice, image and the spoken word. The film is about the experiences of being LGBTQ and emerging from imposed silence to find a voice. During day two of the project, we ran an activity that involved small groups each looking at an example of a stimulus or piece of art, discussing what participants saw in the pieces and what they thought each piece of art might offer in terms of its form and structure. In selecting the art for this session, we chose pieces that used different media, the idea being that every participant would hopefully connect with at least one style, medium or idea and be able to respond to that piece with ideas of their own. We also thought about the ways in which participants might emulate each of the pieces and selected on the basis that we had a reasonable chance of supporting their ideas with resources and staff expertise. We chose not to use artworks which might trigger ideas we couldn't support within the project, so no large-scale metal work sculptures were selected, for example. We used Maya Angelou's spoken word piece *And Still I Rise* (1978), Gillian Wearing's video art piece *2 into 1* (1997), Sam Taylor-Wood's film *Still Life* (2001) and a range of print images of two-dimensional artworks, including Francis Bacon's *Triptych – August 1972*. We set these works up in four corners of the workshop space.

We split the group into four smaller groups and asked them to move to each corner of the room in turn, spending five minutes at each 'station'. In response to this activity, Isaac and Elizabeth, who found themselves in a small group together, began to talk about Gillian Wearing's video work. *2 into 1* shows a mother and her twin sons lip-synching each other's interviews about their family relationship. Wearing's works explore the slippage between private identification and public expression, between those aspects of themselves which people try to hide and those which they are willing or able to reveal. Isaac and Elizabeth both enjoyed the film and spent time after this initial exercise talking about what they liked, what it led them to think about. We had asked people to break into pairs or small groups near the piece of work they liked the most and to re-watch it/re-look at it, and chat to other people who had gathered at that piece of work to talk about it, and to talk about how their own ideas related to gender, sexuality and age might connect with this art form.

Isaac and Elizabeth took inspiration from the concept of creating pathos by 'channelling' one person's voice and experiences through another's body. Both of them wrote a piece of text about their own experiences of being part of a LGBTQ social history. They rehearsed speaking their own texts and then audio recorded themselves speaking the words. They then took each other's audio recordings and writing, and listened and read until they were very familiar with their partner's work. They listened to each other's spoken words on headphones and began trying to speak them out loud, adopting the other person's timing, pace and rhythms of speech as precisely as possible.

Speaking the words of another led them both to process the meaning of another person's words in more engaged ways. Through listening so acutely on headphones, they literally heard the words that were crafted by and important to another person many more times than they would have during a conversation or just by reading one another's words on the page. By speaking another person's words in such a concentrated, conscious way, they began to embody the sentiments of that other.

Using arts as a methodology: can you please all of the people?

In the *INTERarts project*, we used the arts as a method to bring older and younger LGBTQ people together. At the planning stage, the art media initially included photography, video, installations, sound performance and creative writing, although they were expanded to include more traditional arts-based media such as painting to accommodate the interests of older people in particular. When we met some of the older potential participants at the *Opening Doors* groups, some asked if they would be able to paint with oils, for example. Being able to respond to these questions and include other practices in the workshops was of significant importance as we planned a space for the encounters that would offer a variety of cultural opportunities which would allow participants to engage with the arts in ways that were familiar to them, but also to experiment with cultural forms, art practices or technology that were new to them:

> Before the project began, project workers went to recruit potential participants at an older men's and an older women's group. This was an important step in gaining participation from older people as it gave project

workers the opportunity to discuss the project, address any questions, and provide reassurance as to the content of the workshops and the arts based methods. Future intergenerational projects should consider this recruitment strategy, and incorporate this into project planning.

(Kneale et al., 2011, p. 28)

To consider this idea of who participates and who does not, within the Magic Me projects *This is My Life* (2007–2008) and *Pen Friends* (2006–2009) facilitators worked with people who were unable or unwilling to participate in projects outside of their homes (Gilfoy and McAvinchey, 2009; McAvinchey, 2013). Instead of using the term 'housebound', Magic Me refers to people as being 'at home'. This use of language forces a shift away from the idea of an older person being stuck in or bound to a place that is home, outside of the public sphere, and enables us to think more positively about ways of engaging people in the arts when moving or travelling would be barriers to their participation. Applied arts practice frequently engages with the ethics, practicalities and politics of participation. The *INTERarts project* was based outside of people's homes and did require participants to attend workshops at the project venue with specific facilities. The point of good practice taken from the Magic Me examples was about spending time with participants in their own environments where possible during the process of reaching out and inviting people to consider making the commitment to travel, to come to a new place and space, to meet new people. One older lesbian woman who engaged fully with the project commented: "when I first heard about the project, my immediate reaction was:

'[O]h, that's not me', but when I talked to them about it and they said 'of course it's for you, you don't have to be an artist, you can just come and try things out' and that's what I did. [...] I am glad they encouraged me.

(Kneale et al., 2011, p. 44)

On a pragmatic level, in order to support all participants' creative processes and to stimulate them to develop their ideas in ways they might not have considered themselves, we employed a relatively high level of staffing. We brought different facilitators in each week according to the specific workshops we delivered and had four or five project team members working with a group of 16 to 20 participants. Part of the planning for sessions involved ensuring that the staff were spending time with each person, pair or small group throughout the day so that each of the artworks being developed was being fully supported, particularly where participants were using multimedia equipment and software that they hadn't used before.

The use of different media meant that the participants worked in different spaces. Those using video and editing equipment worked around the building as they filmed and then moved into an edit suite to shape the footage. A voice workshop took place in a practical studio space. We had access to multiple spaces and planned the sessions with multiple activities taking place simultaneously, thereby offering choice and variation for participants. We also encouraged participants to work on their ideas development and, latterly, the art pieces, in between workshops. We invited them to request particular resources, so some people took away materials such as pastels and charcoal or cameras and returned them at the following session.

Vald's photography project provides an example of work that gives an insight into how this flexible mode of working enables the creative process. Vald was 86 years of age and identified as a lesbian. She created a piece of work entitled '(How to) Spot a Dyke'. Alongside the photographs she curated, some of which may be seen on the *INTERarts project* website (Gendered Intelligence, 2013), she provided a written commentary and explained how she worked with several different people (participants and project staff) doing a number of specific activities during the workshops, worked alone at times and worked at home:

> Following the first session I decided to concentrate on what I call lesbian signifiers, i.e. things that identify me as a lesbian to anyone who looks at me (especially people I would expect to pick up on these signs). I was paired with Michelle for a photographic project. With the camera we were given we took photos of each other and objects in the space. Michelle took a photo of my right ear with the double women's symbol earring and of my left hand with its pinky ring. We also photographed each other in the mirror of a window. Later Catherine took a photo of my left ear with the labrys (a feminist symbol) earring. I then joined the drawing group and drew a portrait of Syriah while she drew one of me [...] I also drew my left hand. At home I photographed some of the T-shirts I have worn at London Pride and realised that I had been a lesbian in London since I first came out at 35, so it is an important place for me [...] I have also included a photo of me and one of the Age Concern Opening Doors bus at London Pride 2010.
>
> (Vald, 2011)

Some participants reflected that they appreciated the natural way in which bonds between people were allowed to develop. We did not pair people up in older/younger pairs as sometimes happens in intergenerational work. Over one-third of participants (9 of the 26 who participated) reported an improvement in the way they mixed in social situations, which suggests that the project did successfully foster social relations for many involved. Furthermore, both the participants and the project workers reflected that the arts provided a concrete focus which brought people together:

> There was a consensus that bringing people together simply to discuss their issues would not be enough for a project to succeed and the arts theme and the final exhibition gave the project focus.
>
> (Kneale et al., 2011, p. 45)

One of the older participants commented specifically on this point:

> Yes, I think that the art focus is fantastically important and I think that [...] because there is going to be an end product it focuses people and avoids some of the self-consciousness about what we are here for and some of the feelings of slight artificiality you can get in getting people together just to discuss.
>
> (Kneale et al., 2011, pp. 45–46)

Conclusion

The *INTERarts project* was unique in bringing older and younger LGBTQ people together to explore gender, sexuality and ageing. There is some evidence to suggest that older LGBT people are less likely to have children and grandchildren (Guasp, 2011, p. 4). That is, LGBT people are less often part of a traditional family unit and therefore may mix with younger people less. Actually, the *INTERarts project* participants' family backgrounds were varied: one older woman who identified as a lesbian joined the project with her granddaughter, who also identified as a lesbian. There were also participants who did have minimal contact with a family of orientation, and instead spoke of a chosen family or a queer family, meaning people they chose to form close bonds with who were not part of the family in which they had been brought up. One of the project facilitators observed:

> For many people the family environment is a heterosexual set up and so if you are a younger person who is LGBT you are not going to have that kind of conversation with your grandparents, people from different generations and I think there is some value bringing LGBT people together across generations to share some of those exchanges to basically form bonds in the way you do within family life and vice versa.
>
> (Kneale et al., 2011, p. 35)

The project was significant in that it offered opportunities for older and younger LGBTQ people to talk about and share their lived experiences as LGBTQ people, and to bring forth the complex range of experience of gender, age and sexuality among the group.

The model of practice was notable in providing a space for all participants to collaborate and to create art in ways that suited them, while also challenging them to develop new ideas and skills. In deciding against the model of intergenerational work where older people provide stories and younger people create the artistic response, we were inviting stories from all participants and facilitating creative engagement with everyone.

Notes

1 Magic Me is a leading intergenerational arts organisation in the UK. They are based in East London and do work in schools, museums, older people's clubs, care homes, community and cultural organisations.
2 vInspired is the United Kingdom's leading youth volunteering organisation. They facilitate volunteering opportunities that support young people to develop transferable skills. Pfizer is an international biopharmaceutical company that develops medicines, vaccines and consumer health care products. Pfizer have a range of social investment programmes which offer support in the form of financial grants and match funding, for example, to groups and projects which have aims related to well-being and health.

References

Angelou, M. (1978) *And Still I Rise*. New York: Random House.

Asian Arts Agency (2017) Available at http://asianartsagency.co.uk/what-we-do/education/the-desh-project/ (accessed 29 January 2016).

Bacon, F. (1972) *Triptych – August 1972*.

Butler, J. (1997) *Excitable Speech: A Politics of the Performative*. New York: Routledge.

Clarke, E. and Gustafsson Wood, I. (2011) *Queer Voices (INTERarts project)*, Gendered Intelligence. Available at https://interartsproject.wordpress.com/the-exhibition/video/ (accessed 14 December 2015).

Connell, R. (2002) *Gender*. Cambridge: Polity Press.

Elders Share the Arts (2016) *Intergenerational Arts*. Available at www.estanyc.org/core_programs/intergenerational_arts.php (accessed 29 January 2016).

Epstein, A. and Boisvert, C. (2001) 'Let's do something together: Identifying the effective components of intergenerational programmes', *Journal of Intergenerational Relations,* 4(3): 87–109.

Fanning, C. (2016) *Intergenerational Youth Arts Practice – Part 1*. Youth Arts Programme Blog. National Youth Council of Ireland. Available at /www.youtharts.ie/blog/intergenerational-youth-arts-practice-part-1 (accessed 25 January 2016).

Gendered Intelligence and GALYIC (2007) *A Guide for Young Trans People in the UK*. Department of Health.

Gendered Intelligence (2009–2017) Available at www.genderedintelligence.co.uk/projects Accessed 02 December 2015 (accessed 14 December 2015).

Gendered Intelligence (2013) *INTERarts* project website. Available at https://interartsproject.wordpress.com/the-exhibition/photographs-prints-and-paintings/ (accessed 14 December 2015).

Gilfoy, K. and McAvinchey, C. (2009) *Our Generations: Report on a Three Year Programme of Intergenerational Arts Projects in Tower Hamlets, East London*. London: Magic Me.

Greer, S. (2012) *Contemporary British Queer Performance*. Basingstoke: Palgrave Macmillan.

Guasp, A. (2011) Lesbian, Gay and Bisexual People in Later Life. London: Stonewall.

Hatton-Yeo, A. (2006) *Intergenerational Practice in the UK*. Stoke-on-Trent: Beth Johnson Foundation.

House of Commons Women and Equalities Committee (2015) *Transgender Equality Report*. Available at www.parliament.uk/womenandequalities (accessed 20 January 2016).

Houseal, J., Ray, K. and Teitelbaum, S. (2013) 'Identifying, confronting and disrupting stereotypes: Role on the Wall in an intergenerational LGBTQ applied theatre project', *Research in Drama Education: The Journal of Applied Theatre and Performance*, 18(2): 111–119.

Kneale, D., Serra, V., Bamford, S-M. and Diener, L. (2011) *Celebrating Intergenerational Diversity: An Evaluation of Three Projects Working with Younger and Older Lesbian, Gay, Bisexual and Transgender People*. London: International Longevity Centre UK.

Lloyd, J. (2008) *The State of Intergenerational Relations Today: A Research and Discussion Paper*. London: International Longevity Centre UK.

Magic Me (2015) *Frames of Brick Lane*. Available at www.magicme.co.uk/frames/ (accessed 29 January 2016).

McAvinchey, C. (2013) 'Arts practice with older people in private and domestic spaces', *Research in Drama Education: The Journal of Applied Theatre and Performance*, 18(4): 359–373.

McNay, A. and Stewart, J. (2015) 'GI's anatomy: Drawing sex, drawing gender, drawing bodies', *TSQ: Transgender Studies Quarterly*, 2(2): 330–335.

O Connor, A. (2002) *Unwrapping Creativity: An Intergenerational Approach* (Pilot Phase 1998–2001) Sligo. Sligo Arts Office. Available at www.sligoarts.ie/media/SligoArts/Publications/Downloads/The%20Maugherow%20Project_Unwrapping%20Creativity.pdf (accessed 29 January 2016).

Opening Doors London (2014) Available at http://openingdoorslondon.org.uk/ (accessed 14 March 2016).

Perlstein, S. and Bliss, J. (1994) *Generating Community: Intergenerational Partnership through the Expressive Arts*. New York: Elders Share the Arts.

Potter, C., Bamford, SM. and Kneale, D. (2011) *Bridging the Gap: Exploring the Potential for Bringing Older and Younger LGBT People Together: An Evidence Review Examining the Context of Intergenerational Project Work in the LGBT Community*. London: International Longevity Centre UK.

Rooke, A. (2010) 'Trans youth, science and art: Creating (trans) gendered space', *Gender, Place & Culture*, 17(5): 655–672.

Rubin, H. (2003) *Self-made Men: Identity and Embodiment among Transsexual Men*. Nashville: Vanderbilt University Press.

Rubin, SE., Gendron, TL., Wren, CA., Gonzales, EG. and Peron, EP. (2015) 'Challenging gerontophobia and ageism through a collaborative intergenerational art program', *Journal of Intergenerational Relationships*, 13: 241–254.

Sandell, R. (2017) *Museums, Moralities and Human Rights*. London: Routledge.

Springate, I., Atkinson, M. and Martin, K. (2008) *Intergenerational Practice: A Review of the Literature* (LGA Research Report F/SR262). Slough: NFER.

Stryker, S. and Whittle, S. (2006) *The Transgender Studies Reader*. New York: Routledge.

Taylor-Wood, S. (2001) *Still Life*. [Video file.] Available at www.youtube.com/watch?v=36WUgFMDY-M (accessed 11 April 2015).

University Southern California Davis School of Gerentology. (2016) *Zekenim: Honoring and Celebrating Los Angeles' Jewish Elders*. Available at www.zekenim.org/ (accessed 29 January 2016).

Vald. (2011) *(How to) Spot a Dyke*. INTERarts project, Gendered Intelligence. Available at https://interartsproject.wordpress.com/the-exhibition/photographs-prints-and-paintings/ (accessed 13 July 2015).

Valentine, D. (2007) *Imagining Transgender: An Ethnography of a Category*. Durham, NC: Duke University Press.

Wearing, G. (1997) *2 into 1*. [Video file.] Available at www.youtube.com/watch?v=36WUgFMDY-M (accessed 11 April 2015).

Wellcome Collection Blog. (2015) *Transvengers Review and Interview*. Available at http://blog.wellcomecollection.org/2015/04/14/transvengers-youth-review-interview/#more-5979 (accessed 2 February 2016).

Williams, R. (2014) 'Facebook's 71 gender options come to UK users [Online]', *Telegraph Online*. Available at www.telegraph.co.uk/technology/facebook/10930654/Facebooks-71-gender-options-come-to-UK-users.html (accessed 25 January 2016).

10 Fabled and far-off places

The preferred futures of older lesbian and gay adults in long-term care environments

Paul Willis, Michele Raithby and Tracey Maegusuku-Hewett

Introduction

Dedicated long-term care provision for older lesbian, gay and bisexual (LGB) adults is an established and growing phenomenon internationally, for example, LGB (and including transgender)-specific retirement homes are operating in European nations and in some US states (Carr and Ross, 2013; Ross, 2016; Westwood, 2016a). An inherent expectation within this new market is that LGB older adults will receive person-centred, inclusive and sensitive care which recognises non-heterosexual ageing. Within the UK, demands for separate care settings potentially run against the intended objectives of the Equality Act 2010 that requires all service providers in England and Wales, public and private, to provide non-discriminatory services. This begs the question of whether the expansion of specialist provision or the enhancement of existing services for older people should be a future priority for public bodies, LGB advocacy groups and housing providers. In this chapter we explore some of the assumptions and meanings inherent in older adults' discussions about lesbian and gay-specific long-term care as a newly evolving agenda that spans social care, housing and ageing policy. We focus critically on the commentaries provided by a small sample of lesbian- and gay-identifying older adults (50–76 years) about the meaning and significance of gender- and sexuality-specific care environments. We refer to 'lesbian and gay adults' as this more accurately reflects the membership of our interview sample; out of 29 participants only one person identified as bisexual and their interview account is not referenced in this discussion. In some places when discussing other sources we refer to 'LGB' where other authors have included references to bisexual adults in their work. To inform our discussion we present qualitative findings from a mixed-methods study into the provision of long-term care to older lesbian and gay adults in Wales that concluded in 2013 (see Willis et al., 2016).[1] In particular we are interested in the degree of importance which older lesbian and gay adults place on specialist care settings for service users from minority groups, in this context older people located at the socio-sexual margins of UK society. We identify a discourse of community cohesion running throughout older adults' accounts of preferred future care while pointing to nuanced differences in preferences across gender and sexual identity.

Within existing research literature, the preferences of older lesbian and gay adults vary between those advocating for the enhancement of mainstream housing and care, to others arguing for the delivery of specialist housing and aged care services. Emphasis is given to the importance of choice, suggesting the need for a range of mainstream and specialist housing (Westwood, 2016b). Moreover, Westwood (2016a) contends that the lack of both LGB-friendly care home provision and specialist LGB provision represent spatial inequalities for older adults from sexual minority backgrounds. Internationally, preferences for lesbian- and gay-only residential services have likewise been identified in other samples of LGB adults (Barrett, 2008; Health and Care Development Ltd, 2006; Johnson et al., 2005; Jackson et al., 2008; Hughes, 2009; Stein et al., 2010). Within the UK, this is significant in the wake of recent research highlighting social isolation as an acute issue for lesbian and gay older adults. The Stonewall (2011) survey conducted in Great Britain (England, Wales and Scotland) suggests that LGB adults over 55 years are more likely to live alone and less likely to have regular contact with biological family compared to heterosexual peers. In addition, three out of five respondents reported lack of confidence in social care services, including housing, to meet their needs (Stonewall, 2011). This finding diminishes the likelihood of this older cohort accessing social care services.

The shifting policy framework for social care in England and Wales may present new opportunities for innovative provision in housing and long-term care services. The Social Services and Well-being (Wales) Act 2014 and the Care Act 2014 (England) give new emphasis to the co-production of services – the co-development of social care services between user groups and local authority agencies, voluntary agencies and social enterprises that are tailored to the care and support needs of the user group. How this can be realised and resourced in the wake of austerity cuts to social care services for adults is yet to be seen (Ismail et al., 2014). LGB (and 'T') voluntary and community services across England and Wales have equally felt the financial impact of recent austerity measures (Colgan et al., 2014). Arguably these are the organisations that are best placed to initiate co-production activities. Despite this economic backdrop, social care policy in England and Wales has paved the way for innovative developments in service provision that may meet the diverse needs, wishes and social circumstances of older adults, including LGB individuals.

About the research

Between 2011 and 2012 29 older lesbian and gay adults living in Wales participated in semi-structured interviews with members of our research team. Older adults were recruited through self-selection methods of purposive and snowball sampling. Research advertisements were circulated through social groups and networks across Wales (e.g. dining clubs or walking groups) targeted at older lesbians and gay men, and via older people's advocacy networks and organisations. Interviews were conducted in a location of the participant's choice, typically in their home. The interview protocol contained questions exploring preferences for future care arrangements, encompassing both domiciliary (care in the home) and long-term care services. Transcripts were thematically coded in NVivo using an interpretative phenomenological framework whereby the focus was on the participant's understanding of their social environment, present challenges and concerns, and future preferences for social care provision, if required.

The sample contained 19 women and 10 men between the ages of 50 and 76 with a skew towards a 'younger-old' sample with only 6 people over the age of 70. One person identified as a cross-dressing male and bisexual; no other participants indicated bisexual identities, despite our attempts to advertise the study through bisexual communities online. As Jones notes (Chapter 2, this volume), it is difficult to fully explore provision for 'LGB' older people when bisexual older people appear hard to access. Eighteen participants resided in towns and villages while 11 participants lived in larger towns and cities. All participants were White Caucasian with 26 people of British descent. Over half the group (18) held either degrees or higher degrees, reflecting a high level of educational attainment. Below we examine participants' reflections on lesbian and gay-tailored care environments, and the ways in which preferred care arrangements are represented in their discussions of 'ideal care' in the future. First names are pseudonyms nominated by participants.

Findings: Preferred futures among 'our own'

Motivations for seeking lesbian and gay-specific settings and long-term care

When reflecting on the future possibility of requiring social care, participants relayed a number of concerns about how they would be received and treated in long-term care settings. Concerns included having to counteract the recurring presumption of heterosexuality; forced separation from same-sex partners and non-biological kin; and experiencing homophobic and heterosexist commentary from both staff and residents (see Willis et al., 2016). These concerns chime with the reported preferences of other older lesbian and gay individuals in the UK (Westwood, 2016b).

Some lesbians held fears about being 'feminised' through the provision of bodily care and their dread of losing control over self-presentation. Liz (53 years old) and Ruby (51 years old) discussed their concerns about a mutual lesbian friend who had recently moved into a nursing home following an acquired brain injury:

[T]he level of care required can be really major and a lot of issues have arisen out her [friend's] situation, bizarre things, I mean in the early months after her accident, her legs were shaved, and she is your classic hairy dyke, and the family found out that they were shaving her legs as an issue of dignity, and that leads us to wonder, 'Well, when we're elderly, will they come and shave our legs to enable us to be 'dignified'? How much say does one have over these things? And the plucking of eyebrows [...] there are people around her who have raised the issue of plucking her eyebrows as part of this idea of what femininity is.

Fifty-year-old lesbian Nicky wanted her wishes about dress and presentation to be clearly outlined in a care plan: 'So my care plan would be lots of cups of tea, hot baths, and no skirts, no dresses, no tights, no frilly girly stuff, it's got to be solid, butch, because I'm fairly butch.' Akin to these concerns was the presumption of heterosexuality that could accompany older lesbian and gay adults into long-term care:

> I mean, you know, we have moved an enormously long way but I mean it still feels a bit like, you know, if you have to go into a residential home is everybody then going to assume, I mean [sighs] how dare you assume I'm heterosexual, you know? And people still do assume.
>
> (Gillian, 66 years old)

For some participants it was difficult to imagine themselves living in a mainstream care setting. It can be argued that this may be a difficult future for many older adults to envision but for lesbian and gay older people it brings with it concerns about social marginalisation and exclusion. These concerns may reflect the extent to which older lesbian and gay adults perceive themselves to be different from others in their neighbourhood. In his secondary analysis of longitudinal data from the Understanding Society survey and drawing upon a sample of nearly 17,000 older heterosexual and LGBT adults, Green (2016, p. 45) found that LGBT adults were more likely to have feelings of dissimilarity to others, which he proposes could result in 'community severance and being socially excluded'. As stated by Jennifer (58 years old):

> I can't imagine it, I'm certainly not looking forward to it, the whole idea of being in residential care and someone looking after you is not, no one wants to do it, no one wants to be there. Yes, if there's a gay one, I'll go there. Where I won't be considered to be odd, or I won't be as odd as everybody else.

Eleanor (54 years old) elaborated on her wishes not to share the same living environment with other heterosexual women, as she was concerned that their lives were too different from her own lesbian life:

But one thing that I wouldn't like would to be in sheltered accommodation just with heterosexual women because there was a programme on [BBC] Radio 4 about this woman who had gone into sheltered housing but she had nothing in common with the other women, so when they were in the communal area they were all talking about their husbands and their children and she said she just felt totally out of it. I couldn't talk about me at all, and I wouldn't like that, wouldn't like to be a lesbian in a heterosexual home.

The majority of women participants, and one male, sought a mutually supportive future with established friends who made up a significant part of their social network. These older adults spoke about their desire to set up co-housing arrangements with lesbian and gay friends with the intended aim of providing mutual care and support and, if required, employing care staff who suited their needs and preferences; we discuss this in more depth in the next section. Sharing common ties with familiar peers were important dimensions in thinking about future care arrangements that also allayed other fears about discriminatory treatment or the emotional labour of combating heterosexual assumptions. Living in a non-discriminatory environment in which one's sexuality is not under question or perceived outside sexual norms is a standard expectation that should be provided by public and private services under the statutory provisions of the Equality Act 2010 (England and Wales). The concerns relayed by our participants, and other older lesbian and gay individuals (Westwood, 2016b), suggest that the duties enshrined in legislation are yet to fully trickle down into practice and provision.

Fabled and far-off places: the future possibility of lesbian and gay-specific facilities

Over half the sample (13 women, 3 men) indicated a preference to live in specialised facilities targeted towards members of sexual minority groups. Across the findings, there were no discernible patterns based on differences in the age of participants; however, there were evident differences in housing preferences between women and men, as discussed below. Given the number of concerns and anxieties expressed about mainstream care, this finding is not surprising and it mirrors the self-reported preferences of older LGB adults across other nations, including the UK, USA and Australia (Johnson et al., 2005; Jackson et al., 2008; Hughes, 2009; Stein et al., 2010; Westwood, 2016b). Closer to Welsh borders, the 'Gay and Grey in Dorset' project in Southern England surveyed 90 older LGB and transgender people (aged 50–90) and found that respondents preferred 'gay-friendly' homes (38.5%) or 'gay mixed' facilities as future options for care (Health and Care Development Ltd, 2006). A more recent UK-wide mixed method study by Almack et al. (2014) found that almost two-thirds of their 237 survey respondents expressed a preference for 'LGBT'-specific services in old age, and a lack of confidence in mainstream services. There is limited evidence to date on residents' experiences of LGBT-specific settings; however, emerging research indicates positive outcomes for residents, including the expansion of social networks and reported feelings of acceptance and inclusion (Sullivan, 2014).

Threaded throughout participants' discussions about preferred future living environments is a discourse of community cohesion – statements, metaphors and expressions that convey beliefs about idyllic future settings for older lesbian and gay adults and that transmit ideals of social cohesion, harmony and commonality among women communities and lesbian and gay groups. Following the postmodern discussions of Foucault (1990), we use the term 'discourse' in reference to linguistic systems of language and representation that produce what social actors perceive as social reality – the sociocultural lens that determines what seems possible or tangible, and equally, unobtainable (McHoul and Grace, 1997). To a certain extent participants are personally invested in this discourse but equally recognise that these future possibilities are blurred and unsubstantiated, and are not without limitations in delivering a good quality of life in later years. Lesbian- and gay-specific facilities were framed as 'ideal' settings that participants perceived as a potential reality but possibly not to be fully realised in their lifetime. In this context, specialist residential settings were perceived to be part-reality, part-fantasy. Angela (65 years old) discussed her 'fantasised' plan about being part of a women's collective 'lesbians of the purple rinse' which she had created with her friends:

> We've all sat down and fantasised about having the lesbian home and people have talked about buying houses with stables that could be turned into individual rooms and I actually have a pact with somebody about when I finally get to accept that I'm old I'll have a purple rinse. I am quite fond of purple anyway, but that will be the moment, I will go 'okay I'm old' and have a purple rinse, and that's what we're going to do, we're going to be lesbians of the purple rinse!

Participants made occasional references to 'rumoured' developments in bigger cities across England such as London and Manchester but without concrete details. Others recalled sighting media reports about lesbian- and gay-specific facilities in European nations such as Germany, the Netherlands and Spain, all national contexts far removed from their social and geographical environments in Wales:

> Cos it was interesting in our last edition of the Women's [community newsletter] there was a note at the back to say that Spain are to get the first LGB care home for the elderly, well I was quite interested by that, a group of elderly Spanish gay men rebelling against the homophobia of a generation by setting up the country's first lesbian and gay retirement home.
>
> (Amy, 58 years old)

James (63 years old) compared his ideal vision for supported living to the fictional household of '28 Barbary Lane' featured in Armistead Maupin's *Tales of the City* novels about an eccentric landlady and her diverse lodgers living in the urban heart of San Francisco:

> I suppose you know about 28 Barbary Lane, do you? Like I haven't missed a book, they're about a household in San Francisco, a number of them and the owner of the household, it's fiction, right, but there's quite a bit of, the owner of the household is transgender, Mrs Madrigal, was a man, and she's got all these alternative people living in her flats, it's based on a lot of things that have happened there, you know, people have come together and I'm not ruling that out as we need to help each other as a gay community, you know, yeah, that's a bit far-fetched isn't it really.

While describing his vision as 'far-fetched', James draws upon the fictional composition of individual lodgers from socially (and sexually) diverse backgrounds living harmoniously under one roof as a metaphorical cornerstone for articulating his preferred living arrangements.

Previous experiences of social cohesion and connection in lesbian and gay social groups formed the basis for some participants' preferences for seeking similar environments in long-term care. Amy (58 years old) sought a social climate similar to the 'feeling in the air' she had previously felt at lesbian and gay social events. While difficult to articulate, the feeling described by her suggests an atmosphere of affirmation and validation:

> [I]t's like on Saturday night we had a women's own gay disco down [Welsh town], and that was a great feeling, like the women-only tea dance, that was just a great feeling really and I think that you know if it were to happen in an ideal world a gay care home would have that same feeling I think and there'd be no questioning of sexuality particularly like there might be in a normal care home and/or discrimination then because of your sexuality.

Other participants likewise emphasised the importance of commonality and connection – seeking shared living arrangements with 'other people like me'. Within participants' accounts there was an intrinsic assumption that lesbian and gay elders share common characteristics and interests which can provide the basis for communal living:

> "Okay, I make assumptions about everybody and with gay men and lesbians I make an assumption that we are going to find it easier to communicate with each other, because I assume we're going to have things in common, we're going to have life experiences in common [...] I'm more certain about that when I first meet them than I am about

straight people, it's just a prejudice I've got. Yes, it is based on experience, I suppose.

(Mary, 61 years old)

Several women recounted their vision of communal living with other lesbians from their own social networks in which care would be provided on a mutual basis with the option of procuring formal care services:

And on a couple of occasions over the past five to six years, I've got friends, and I've come across some house with a cottage-type complex for sale and we've emailed each other and thought, 'Could three or four of us sell our properties and invest in somewhere like this and we could all live together with each other?' And it tends to go a bit wrong because it's the wrong location for somebody to go and visit their children, or their grandchildren. But I think it's a fairly common fantasy.

(Liz, 53 years old)

Similarly, Nick elaborated on the conversations he had with his friends about investing in shared living under the same roof and eventually over time collectively buying in care provision:

[N]one of my friends have had to go into homes so far, we're all well and able to look after ourselves but we've talked very often about buying a house and so the first person to go into the house, we would all gradually move in there and all look after each other in a situation, and I think a few of us are pretty serious about that and if there was a financial arrangement then I would go with that and live in a sort of a community and as long as it was on the coast.

(Nick, 60 years old)

These envisioned futures may not be realised for all lesbian and gay older people for whom research suggests that while they may have slightly more friends than their heterosexual peers, these friends are also more likely to live at a distant proximity, and so do not provide a compensatory factor for limited or no kinship ties (Green, 2016). This may mean that many lesbian and gay adults are more reliant on formal social care provision.

Intersection of gender and sexuality: lesbians seeking women-only spaces

Using an intersectional approach, other scholars in sexuality and ageing studies have sought to trouble the representation of older LGB adults as a homogenised group that share the same, too often essentialised, characteristics (Cronin and King, 2010). Intersectional approaches within LGB studies more broadly are concerned with the intersections of difference that produce different patterns and outcomes of inequality for different groups clustered under the loosely demarcated category of 'LGB' and the intersections that shape political activism and processes among LGB interest groups (Fish, 2008). For example, Moore's (2010) research with Black lesbian and gay activists in the USA points to their negotiation of oppositional identities and social distancing by members of both 'communities' who perceive inconsistencies in their identity allegiances. The 'LGB community' is not an inclusive place for all and, with limited knowledge about older bisexual adults' social networks, we do not have a basis for understanding how bisexual adults experience these community settings. In another Welsh study, we found that among lesbian and gay adults with mental health issues, older males perceived LGB-specific spaces, such as online communities and social events, to be highly sexualised and ageist spaces from which they felt excluded (Maegusuku-Hewett et al., 2014). Furthermore, older lesbians report experiences of discrimination across three intersecting axes: homophobia, ageism and sexism (Averett et al., 2013), and may be equally subject to sexist assumptions within gay male communities. In our analysis, accounting for gendered differences in older lesbian and gay adults' preferences is a way of recognising how gender can lend different shades of meaning to the importance of community and shared identity for lesbians. These are women who may have lived a significant part of their life histories invisible, for some hidden in heterosexual marriages and, prior to the arrival of equal opportunity laws from 2003 onward in the UK, not recognised or protected by political and social institutions. While these women's relationships were not subject to criminal sanctions, they have still experienced significant social sanctions. In this historical context gender matters, and it mattered more so for 14 older women in the sample who stated a definite preference for women-only residential communities and care settings. But the degree to which sexual identity and gender mattered shifted across the group of women participating in our study. For some, gender-specific settings were a greater priority while for others lesbian-only spaces were the ideal. The weight given to 'community' and its meaning varied. In the following, Mary (61 years old) asserts a strong position for lesbian-only spaces:

> I mean when we were much younger we [partner and I] had a dream with these various other lesbian couple friends of ours, there were about eight of us, and we were going to buy this big house and we were going to have young lesbians to come and be our carers. [...] Oh in our little dream, we had a big estate with a house and the nursing bit and we had separate little houses as well and we had all these young dykes coming to look after us [laughter]. I'd like an old dyke's home thank you!

Likewise, Eleanor (54 years old) advocated lesbian sheltered accommodation but simultaneously labelled this future plan as unrealistic and 'pie in the sky' thinking:

> It's more understanding isn't it, because my ideal in terms of care would be to be in a sort of sheltered accommodation that was just for lesbians, but I'm not sure we agree, but that would be me because I wouldn't particularly want men around, to be honest, gay men or straight men, I'd want to be in a women-only environment, preferably a lesbian one. That's probably pie in the sky.

Sarah (59 years old) expressed her wishes for female (preferably lesbian) carers in whom trust and confidence in the intimate care being provided would be paramount:

> [A]nd again I think it is about a woman, somebody of the same sex, I wouldn't want a man coming in to give care. I know when we went into the hospital to see your [partner's] mum there was a man taking your mum to the toilet and I just wouldn't want that. I'm sure that's the same with a lot of women, it's not just a lesbian thing, it's about just feeling more secure with another woman as opposed to a man, that's important, but it's about trusting them isn't it, it's about trusting somebody to be absolutely okay with who you are.

The enthusiasm for women-only care settings was driven by several factors: first, the desire to be among other residents and staff where there was lived experience and understanding of being in relationships with other women; second, concerns about sharing living environments with older men, which was unfamiliar, and in some cases unwelcome, territory; and third, unease about the prospect of receiving intimate care from male staff. Life history is an important facet here in recognising that some lesbians have invested a significant period of their lives in predominantly women-only networks and communities. Women's groups and networks have been a central organising feature for many lesbians living in the UK in late modernity (Traies, 2015; Wilkins, 2016).

It is important to distinguish variations in lesbians' reported preferences for women-only environments. Similarly in other international studies lesbians have reported a preference for purpose-built retirement homes shared with older women, regardless of sexual identity (Phillips and Marks, 2006). One participant, Olwen (72 years old), stipulated her wish for a feminist environment in which shared feminist beliefs and values among women residents held greater importance than a specific lesbian space. Other women, including Gillian and Gwenno, indicated their preference for women-only facilities – sexual identity was a less significant dimension for these women while gender-specific spaces remained paramount to their quality of life:

> I mean [sighs] I mean it's difficult in a sense because everybody probably has different needs. Some people are quite happy to have, or might be quite happy to have a lesbian and gay and bisexual and transsexual

set-up, you know, that's on its own as it were. Other people like me would actually feel much happier in a women-only set-up, regardless of whether they're lesbian or not.

(Gillian, 66 years old)

I was thinking on reflection that as far as I'm concerned if I were contemplating living in these care establishments, I think gender is more important to me than sexuality and I think I would want to be in a female or female-friendly set-up, rather than be with gay men, say. It sounds very forbidding but I just think day-by-day I would not want to live in a mixed gender home.

(Gwenno, 75 years old)

A small group of women were receptive to the possibility of lesbian and gay-only settings in which affiliation with lesbian and gay identities trumped the prospect of residing in mainstream care settings. Karin (54 years old) specified a clear order of preference, the first being lesbian-only followed by lesbian and gay-only facilities:

Cos if I had to go into a care home, I'd definitely prefer a lesbian care home, failing that lesbian and gay, absolutely and your basic bog standard mixed care home would be awful so I'd much rather have the suicide van and that option.

Recognising the cracks and fissures in ideal settings

Present in participants' reflections on future care were moments of recognition that neither sexuality- nor gender-specific settings could meet all individuals' social needs and requirements under the broad, and arguably nebulous, LGB umbrella. These points of recognition represent cracks and fissures in the discourse of community cohesion, as outlined above. This illustrates how this discourse is by no means totalising or a complete picture of lesbian and gay individuals' lives, particularly when accounting for intersecting differences in gender. Several participants were mindful that sharing the same affiliation with lesbian and gay identities did not guarantee commonality or social cohesion among group members, as acknowledged by Angela (65 years old): "but there's just no guarantee that you're going to get on with other lesbians but at least they kind of understand a lot more." Angela further comments on different identities within lesbian women's groups: "Not that long ago we [lesbian women] had separate identities, we weren't all bunched together in one string, and there is a difference, we have cultural difference, we're not all one bunch." Participants' accounts conveyed a degree of self-reflexivity – recognising one's socially situated status within a sexual minority group and the cohesion it purportedly brings while also acknowledging how these assumptions may not translate into lived reality. Mary (61 years old) reflected on her assumptions about group cohesion among lesbian and gay groups:

> Okay, I make assumptions about everybody and with gay men and lesbians I make an assumption that we are going to find it easier to communicate with each other that we are going to, because I assume we're going to have things in common, we're going to have life experiences in common, I just assume that we're going to get on with each other, and I'm more certain about that when I first meet them than I am about straight people.

Similarly, Paul (53 years old) acknowledged the potential challenges of bringing disparate gay and lesbian individuals together with very different personalities and characteristics: "And I think we do all sort of come together but we're very different aren't we, personalities and types, so it's a little bit of a, it's not an artificial distinction is it." Colin (66 years old) expressed his scepticism about setting up 'gay-only' facilities which he perceived as potentially having a ghetto effect in separating older lesbian and gay adults from wider communities:

> I mean there have been previous initiatives and most of them have floundered; either they never got off the ground cos there was no long-term finance, mostly financial problems, yeah. I certainly, it certainly wouldn't be my primary aim to have a separate sort of gay ghetto for the care situation, no.

Others stated concerns about the future affordability of specialised facilities – lesbian- and gay-specific or gender-specific housing and residential care were perceived to be potentially costly and limited to primarily wealthier lesbians and gay men with high-bracket incomes:

> But I realise in fact that I'd never be able to afford to be part of one of those anyway, because you're paying extra for the shared part and of course my address is a bit confusing really in a way, although I live in the east of the city, it's not where most other people I know live because it's a very working-class area really, but that's just about my income really, so I don't know whether I'd have enough money for a nice older person's home anyway, I might have whatever's left over. [...] So yeah, old people's home, gay staff [laughs]. Where are these millionaire gay men that can make this happen?! So that's the ideal that's not going to happen.
>
> (Margaret, 66 years old)

Mary (61 years old) sought an "old dyke's home" for when she and her partner were older and had additional care needs. However the current state of the economy and finite financial resources weighed on her mind:

> Oh that's a fear, that the money would run out, which it would and then the whatever care would be inadequate I mean by the time me and [partner] are old enough to be needing other people to care for us the economy will be in such a terrible state.

For these participants this social divide made the prospect of lesbian- and gay-specific settings far less tangible, highlighting how class and socioeconomic status shape what participants consider to be realistic and feasible. For some this 'reality check' may diminish the future possibility of living in LGB-specific accommodation.

Implications for future service provision and research

In this chapter we have focused on the voices of older lesbian and gay adults from interview data to canvass their future preferences for long-term care provision if required in their later years. The findings presented add further weight to a growing body of literature detailing the preferences and wishes of older LGBT adults for sexuality- and gender-specific long-term care settings. This evidence of user demand lies within a service vacuum in which there are currently next to no choices about specialist care and housing services for older lesbian and gay adults in the UK. Arguably, the economic realities of austerity measures make the possibility of public service funding, from central and local governments, highly doubtful. The findings we have presented are illuminating on two interrelated bases: first, through the variations in preferred care settings and arrangements across a small sample; second, the fertile ground this presents for exploring co-design and co-production of specialist living facilities that meet individual and small-group needs. The nuanced differences in preferences across this group disrupt the discourse of commonality and community cohesion attached to lesbian and gay identities, and reinforce the importance of investment in multiple models of provision across the social care and housing sector. Participants' descriptions of preferred futures also hint at a range of possibilities for co-producing different models of housing provision, including the support of housing co-operatives among established groups and networks of older lesbians and gay men. Housing providers and social enterprises are well situated to further explore and support these alternative models under the auspices of co-production currently championed in social care policy.

The subtitle of this edited volume, *Minding the Knowledge Gaps*, is pertinent because there are currently two major gaps in the area of housing and social care provision for older lesbian and gay adults. The first gap is robust survey data that captures the varying needs and preferences of this group in later life, particularly among older-old people over 80 years of age. There is an ever-expanding cluster of qualitative, small-scale studies that do not fully encompass the wide variation in preferences for future housing and social care; we locate our own study in this cluster. The second gap is in-depth investigation of self-initiated housing options among existing networks of lesbians and gay men, and a wider gap in addressing those among networks of bisexual adults, as noted previously and elsewhere in this volume. More attention needs to be given to what already works well among lesbian and gay households and shared living arrangements. Key learning from these living arrangements may be transferred to older lesbians and gay men at risk of social exclusion because of increasing health care needs or because of diminished social networks and risk of social isolation. A paramount question for researchers in ageing, social policy makers and service providers is how seemingly idyllic supportive living arrangements initiated in other nations can be made a reality for older lesbian and gay individuals in the UK. Case study research of the growing number of specialist settings within Western European nations, Australia and the United States would be of value in addressing this question. It would also be prudent to examine when specialist initiatives in other nations are unsuccessful and lead to closure – lessons about the rise and decline of such initiatives are equally illuminating.

Note

1 This research was funded by the National Institute for Social Care and Health Research (NISCHR), Welsh Government. The project received ethical approval from the NHS Wales National Research Ethics Service (Reference 11/WA/0217), local R&D approval from Abertawe Bro Morgannwg, Cardiff and Vale and Betsi Cadwaladr University Health Boards, and University ethics approval.

References

Almack, K., Yip, A., Seymour, J., Sargeant, A., Patterson, A. and Makita, M. (2014) *The Last Outing: Exploring End of Life Experiences and Care Needs in the Lives of Older LGBT People*. University of Nottingham. Available at www.nottingham. ac.uk/research/groups/ncare/documents/projects/srcc-project-report-last-outing. pdf.

Averett P., Yoon, I. and Jenkins, CL. (2013) 'Older lesbian experiences of homophobia and ageism', *Journal of Social Service Research,* 39(1): 3–15.

Barrett, C. (2008). *My People: A Project Exploring the Experiences of Gay, Lesbian, Bisexual, Transgender and Intersex Seniors in Aged-care Services.* Available at www.matrixguildvic.org.au/MyPeopleReport2008.pdf.

Carr, S. and Ross, P. (2013) *Assessing Current and Future Housing and Support Options for Older LGB People.* York: Joseph Rowntree Foundation. Available at www.jrf. org.uk/report/assessing-current-and-future-housing-and-support-options-older-lgb-people.

Colgan, F., Hunter, C. and McKearney, A. (2014) *'Staying Alive': The Impact of 'Austerity Cuts' on the LGBT Voluntary and Community Sector (VCS) in England and*

Wales. A TUC Funded Research Report. London: London Metropolitan University. Available at www.tuc.org.uk/sites/default/files/StayingAlive.pdf.

Cronin, A. and King, A. (2010) 'Power, inequality and identifications: Exploring diversity and intersectionality amongst older LGB adults', *Sociology* 44(5): 876–892.

Fish, J. (2008) 'Navigating Queer Street: Researching the intersections of lesbian, gay, bisexual and trans (LGBT) identities in health research', *Sociological Research Online*, 13(1): 1–11. Available at www.socresonline.org.uk/13/1/12.html.

Foucault, M. (1990) *The History of Sexuality: Volume 1: An Introduction*. New York: Vintage Books.

Green, M. (2016) 'Do the companionship and community networks of older LGBT adults compensate for weaker kinship networks', *Quality in Ageing,* 17(1): 36–49.

Health and Care Development Ltd (2006) *Lifting the Lid on Sexuality and Ageing: A Research Project into the Needs, Wants, Fears and Aspirations of Older Lesbians and Gay Men*. Bournemouth: Help and Care.

Hubbard, R. and Rossington, J. (1995) *As We Grow Older: A Study of the Housing and Support Needs of Older Lesbians and Gay Men*. London: Polari. Available at www.openingdoorslondon.org.uk/resources/As_We_Grow_Older.pdf.

Hughes, M. (2009) 'Lesbian and gay people's concerns about ageing and accessing services', *Australian Social Work,* 62(2): 186–201.

Ismail, S., Thorlby, R. and Holder, H. (2014) *Quality Watch Focus On: Social Care for Older People: Reductions in Adult Social Services for Older People in England*. London: The Health Foundation and Nuffield Trust. Available at www.qualitywatch.org.uk/focus-on/social-care-older-people.

Jackson, NC., Johnson, MJ. and Roberts, R. (2008) 'The potential impact of discrimination fears of older gays, lesbians, bisexuals and transgender individuals living in small- to moderate-sized cities on long-term health care', *Journal of Homosexuality,* 54(3): 325–339.

Johnson, MJ., Jackson, NC., Arnette, JK. and Koffman, SD. (2005) 'Gay and lesbian perceptions of discrimination in retirement care facilities', *Journal of Homosexuality*, 49(2): 83–102.

Maegusuku-Hewett, T., Raithby, M. and Willis, P. (2014) 'Life in the Pink Dragon's Den: Mental Health Services and social inclusion for LGBT people in Wales', in Fish, J. and Kaban, K. (eds), *Lesbian, Gay, Bisexual and Trans Health Inequalities: International Perspectives in Social Work*. Bristol: Policy Press.

McHoul, A. and Grace, W. (1997) *A Foucault Primer: Discourse, Power and the Subject*. New York: New York University Press.

Moore, MD. (2010) 'Articulating a politics of (multiple) identities: LGBT sexuality and inclusion in black community life', *Debois Review,* 7(2): 315–334.

Phillips, J. and Marks, G. (2006) 'Coming out, coming in: How do dominant discourses around aged care facilities take into account the identities and needs of ageing lesbians?', *Gay and Lesbian Issues and Psychology Review,* 2(2): 67–77.

Ross, P. (2016) 'Learning from international experiences: Developing older LGBT affirmative housing and care options in England', *Quality in Ageing and Older Adults,* 17(1): 60–70.

Stein, GL., Beckerman, NL. and Sherman, PA. (2010) 'Lesbian and gay elders and long-term care: Identifying the unique psychosocial perspectives and challenges', *Journal of Gerontological Social Work*, 53: 421–435.

Stonewall (2011) *Lesbian, Gay and Bisexual People in Later Life*. London: Stonewall. Available at www.stonewall.org.uk/documents/lgb_in_later_life_final.pdf.

Sullivan, K.M. (2014) 'Acceptance in the domestic environment: The experience of senior housing for lesbian, gay, bisexual, and transgender seniors', *Journal of Gerontological Social Work,* 57(2–4): 235–250.

Traies, J. (2012) '"Women like that": Older lesbians in the UK', in Ward, R., Rivers, I. and Sutherland, M. (eds), *Lesbian, Gay, Bisexual and Transgender Ageing: Biographical Approaches for Inclusive Care and Support.* London: Jessica Kingsley, pp. 67–80.

Traies, J. (2015) 'Old lesbians in the UK: Community and friendship', *Journal of Lesbian Studies,* 19(1): 35–49.

Westwood, S. (2016a) 'LGBT ageing in the UK: Spatial inequalities in older age housing/care provision', *Journal of Poverty and Social Justice,* 24(1): 63–76.

Westwood, S. (2016b) '"We see it as being heterosexualised, being put into a care home": Gender, sexuality and housing/care provision among older LGB individuals in the UK', *Health and Social Care in the Community,* 24(6): 155–163.

Wilkins, J. (2016) 'The significance of affinity groups and safe spaces for older lesbians and bisexual women: Creating support networks and resisting heteronormativity in older age', *Quality in Ageing and Older Adults,* 17(1): 26–35.

Willis, P., Maegusuku-Hewett, T., Raithby, M. and Miles, P. (2016) 'Swimming upstream: The provision of inclusive care to older lesbian, gay and bisexual (LGB) adults in residential and nursing environments in Wales', *Ageing and Society,* 36(2): 282–306.

11 'I didn't come out to go back in the closet'

Ageing and end-of-life care for older LGBT people

Kathryn Almack[1]

You matter because you are you, and you matter to the end of your life.
Dame Cicely Saunders (1918–2005)
(Saunders, 1976)

Introduction

This chapter addresses a particular gap in knowledge concerning the end-of-life care needs and experiences in the lives of older LGBT people. This adds to a more general body of research which has focused on ageing and the broader health and social care issues for older LGBT people (albeit this has primarily focused on gay men's and lesbian health and social care needs).

The chapter provides a brief overview of end-of-life care in England and Wales, and then addresses issues relating to end-of-life care for older LGBT people and the gaps in our knowledge in this area. We then draw upon findings from the first major UK study of end-of-life care needs and experiences in the lives of older LGBT people. Our main focus here is to highlight and discuss concerns identified relating to care at home and support from family and friends that respondents envisaged being able to call upon towards the end of life in the UK. Our findings suggest that diverse needs are not being met or not offering adequate provision for older LGBT people. However, we are also able to highlight positive examples to suggest ways forward to develop equitable service provision that addresses core principles of dignity and respect for all.

Introduction to end-of-life care in England and Wales

Rapid demographic changes (which include ageing populations and more people living with the effects of serious chronic illness towards the end of life) present a pressing public health challenge related to the care and quality of life of older people (Hall et al., 2011). There are 14.9 million people in the UK aged 60 and above (ONS, 2015); using a commonly cited estimate that about 5 to 7 per cent of the population identify as LGBT, that suggests an estimated population of between 745,000 and 1,043,000 LGBT people aged 60 and over in the UK.[2]

In the UK, there is general agreement that the definition of 'end-of-life care' means 'the last year of life'; although it is acknowledged that the period in which such care is needed ranges from a few years to a matter of months, weeks or days, and into bereavement (NHS England, 2014). The UK is an acknowledged leader in palliative and end-of-life care.[3] In 2008, the first-ever English End of Life Care Strategy was launched (DoH, 2008a). This sought to promote high-quality care for all adults at the end of life in England by providing people with more choice about where they would like to live and die. Similar strategies for the end of life have also been developed in Wales, Scotland and Northern Ireland. Consultation for the English End of Life Care Strategy Equality Impact Assessment (DoH, 2008b) noted that in terms of quality of end-of-life care, LGBT people were most at risk of discrimination. The Strategy and the National End of Life Care Programme (2008 to 2013, charged with the implementation of the Strategy) generated significant momentum and improvements in end-of-life care (Kennedy et al., 2009, NHS England, 2014). Actions for End of Life Care: 2014–2016 (NHS England, 2014) reviews these achievements and sets out NHS England's commitments to 'align it with current needs of the population and the changing health and social care landscape' (p. 5). This document identifies that inequalities in end-of-life care for certain groups of people remain; however, LGBT people are conspicuous in their absence in this document – those named are homeless people; black and minority ethnic populations; people with learning disabilities and people with dementia. Most recently, the English Care Quality Commission (CQC, 2016) published a report highlighting continuing inequalities in end-of-life care for people from certain groups, including LGBT people. The report suggests that LGBT people may sometimes experience poorer quality care at the end of their lives because providers do not always understand or fully consider their needs.

Background to LGBT palliative and end-of-life care research

Both evidence of and identifying ways to address inequalities facing LGBT people has been hampered by the dearth of research with a specific focus on older LGBT people's end-of-life care needs and experiences; both as people coming towards the end of life and as carers of partners or friends coming to the end of life.

Harding and colleagues' (2012) systematic review of peer-reviewed research (published between 1990 and 2010) into palliative and end-of-life care in LGBT populations identified only 12 relevant papers (the criteria excluded papers not published in English). The majority of papers resulted from studies in the USA, and the primary focus of the research was found to be end-of-life care relating to cancer in populations of lesbian women and gay men. Again, bisexual (and transgender) people's experiences were notable in their absence. However, this is now a burgeoning field of research. Since Harding et al.'s systematic review which included papers up until 2010, there have been a number of other papers published specifically addressing LGBT experiences and concerns relating to dying, death and bereavement. The bulk of the research comes from Australia, Canada, the USA and the UK. Examples include Almack et al. (2010); Cartwright et al. (2012); Rawlings (2012), and Lawton et al. (2013)

Older people are now the largest group requiring end-of-life care; the majority of deaths in the UK are people over the age of 65 (Ruth and Verne, 2010). While some of the end-of-life care issues facing LGBT older adults are similar to all older people, research is now identifying separate issues that need to be addressed for older LGBT people entering their later and final years of life. Overall there is a lack of understanding of the heterogeneous needs of 'older people', particularly those living in non-traditional family forms. Research in the areas of palliative and end-of-life care have traditionally had a primary focus on family relationships biased towards families (Manthorpe, 2003). An additional consideration for LGBT people is that as LGBT people grow older, there is evidence that they are more at risk of life-threatening conditions where incidence increases with age. These factors can be related to risk behaviours such as smoking or alcohol abuse, which in turn may be attributed to minority stress. Minority stress is a term used to define chronically high levels of stress faced by members of stigmatised minority groups. This may include experiences of stigma, marginalisation or discrimination, now acknowledged as social determinants of health, which may have a significant impact upon the health and well-being of LGBT people (Wilkinson and Marmot, 2003). Minority stress may also contribute to reduced social participation and engagement within society, and delaying or not seeking care because of past experiences or anticipation of facing discrimination. Over their lifetime, LGBT people may avoid preventive health care because of concerns related to both discrimination and insensitivity by health care providers (Almack, 2016).

The study

The data presented in this chapter are drawn from a UK-wide study The Last Outing: Exploring end of life experiences and care needs in the lives of older LGBT people (2012–2015), funded by the Marie Curie Research Programme under a call for proposals addressing the research theme 'variation in care at end of life'. It was a mixed methods study, incorporating a survey (n = 237) and in-depth interviews with a sub-sample of the survey participants (n = 60). The survey was open to people living in the UK aged 60 or over and who self-identified under the umbrella labels of L, G, B and/ or T. We also included LGBT people aged under 60 but in a relationship with a L, G, B and/or T person aged 60 or older. To capture the extent and level of engagement with the topic area of end-of-life care, we asked that participants had some experience of thinking/talking/planning for or receiving end-of-life care, or caring for a same-sex partner or LGBT friend at end of life. We made the survey available online or as a hard copy that we posted out to people with a SAE for return. We recruited participants across the whole of the UK via the research team's extensive LGBT networks; publicity in social and printed media, advertising via generic organisations for older people (retirement organisations, union retirement networks, walking clubs and so on).

The survey included 81 questions (mostly closed questions and scaling of opinions but with some options for further information and some 'open' questions). In addition to demographic and self-identification data, topics covered included the extent to which individuals were open about their sexual orientation and/or gender identity in different settings; questions about health and well-being; about experiences of receiving health and social care oneself or in current or previous caring situations/relationships; ageing; plans and preferences for future care and designating next of kin; and on finances and resources. We draw in part of these data in this chapter to provide a descriptive context of the range of circumstances and experiences of participants. The interview data were analysed via thematic readings; as a research team we identified 8 key themes,[4] and a coding framework (74 items) was then developed, tested and then applied to all 60 interviews. In this chapter we draw upon three key themes: accessibility to help and support at current age; experiences within health and social care settings (for oneself or as a carer); and preferences for how services should be organised. In returning to these themes, we have examined the data for storied accounts (Plummer, 2007), which sensitises us to the contexts within which stories may emerge as well as the societal context (across a life course) that enables some stories to be told and widely heard while others are 'weaker' in this sense of being less widely told and heard.

'Old' LGBT age and end-of-life care

The last major academic study relating to LGBT ageing in the UK was undertaken in 2001/2003 (Heaphy et al., 2003). This study found that meanings attached to ageing and 'old age' by lesbians, gay men and bisexuals was as varied and context-dependent as one might expect to find in the wider culture. Nevertheless, the authors suggested that sexual orientation was relevant in shaping how one sees oneself and is seen by others. LGBT people aged 50 and over were reported to describe themselves as 'older' when referring to their sexual identities and lifestyles. A decade or so later, our pilot work suggested that 50 seemed too 'young' to be included in our study. Stonewall undertook a survey of later life experiences of LGB people in 2011, including those aged 55 and over. Defining later life or old age is problematic and across the developed world a range of chronological ages from 50 to 70 are used to determine 'old age' (Victor, 2010).

Our study had a greater emphasis on end-of-life care than Heaphy et al. (2003) or Stonewall (2011) and it is acknowledged that end-of-life care needs are most common among older age groups (whether as patients or as carers) (Ruth and Verne, 2010) and that older age groups were perhaps more likely to have had cause (for example, through ill-health or through the experience of deaths of people close to them) to reflect more on their own mortality. For the purposes of our study we thus proposed to include people aged 60 or over (but also those under 60 if in a partnership with someone aged 60 or over). Reaching an age where participants or their partners required assistance towards the end of life, or where they had thoughts about an anticipated loss of independence, brought issues about care preferences in later life and towards the end of life into sharp focus.

Home

In relation to end-of-life care, the most commonly expressed option found in surveys conducted about preferences for place of care towards the end of life is to be cared for at home (Gomes and Higginson, 2008; Leadbeater and Garber, 2010). As Pollock discusses, such survey findings are problematic for a number of reasons: the context and framing of questions can influence responses; often people do not specify a preference and/or there is rarely an option for 'it depends' or 'does not matter' (Pollock, 2015).

However, given that 'home' is nevertheless a commonly expressed anticipated place of care and was a preference noted by many of our interview participants (regardless of how achievable this might be), this presented particular anxieties for our participants in a number of ways; not least that home may represent a private, most often 'safe' space to be totally oneself. Opening up previously private domestic settings to wider scrutiny can be daunting, yet more often than not the preference to die at home can necessitate the need to have a range of health and social care professionals coming into one's home and 'coming out to care' (Brotman et al., 2007; Price, 2010):

> If people, carers, are coming into your home, just an acknowledgement about your sexuality and your relationships in the past and things like that and like if you've got a photo of you and your partner out, you don't need to be worried, do you know what I mean.
>
> (Trevor, gay man, aged 54, with older partner)

For many, whose life experiences have included hiding their same-sex relationships, these represent considerations that impact upon feeling safe in accessing home care services. It includes facing scenarios at times when they are likely to feel particularly vulnerable, such as decisions about hiding items associated with one's sexual orientation or gender identity; what or how much information to disclose, or outing oneself to every visiting professional with associated further loss of privacy. There are also understandable fears about discriminatory attitudes, which individuals may feel too vulnerable or dependent on care services to be able to challenge (see Bristowe et al., 2018).

Trans people can face further dilemmas. Service providers often have even less knowledge about the issues relating to trans people than those relating to LGBT individuals and it is important to separate out sexual orientation from gender identity. Trans people can face particular challenges if they have to negotiate intimate care with care workers who may not be aware of their particular needs:

> I've always been very private. As a male to female trans (person) I still having beard growth, this would be an area of care I'd need and want to continue if I am became incapacitated [...] unable to shave and apply hair growth inhibitor myself. And other intimate care – dilation and routine douching to keep the vagina clear of possible infections. Hormone therapy is necessary until death and I'd want that to continue.
>
> (Survey response, anonymous)

It is important to be aware of the diversity among trans people; some will have spent most of their lives with a gender identity and body other than the one assigned at birth, while for others this may be a relatively recent transition.

The above quote indicates someone who described themselves as 'private' – possibly guarded and reticent about being open about their particular care routines. Others may not have undergone any form of gender reassignment surgery. This can lead to feeling apprehensive about revealing one's body to care workers:

> Every time I need bodily care I constantly have to explain my anatomical differences to new people. I'm really worried about going into a care home. My GP, meaning to be kind, said once you go into a care home you become genderless but that is not reassuring.
>
> (Survey response, anonymous)

A trans person's medical records can be inconsistent; one trans woman facing a terminal diagnosis recalled how this was dealt with sensitively by staff:

> I was in hospital and somebody came along and drew the curtains and I thought oh shit what's going on. She was the ward secretary or something and she said "I'm having problems matching up your file because you say you've had [name of condition] but we've got no record. The nearest we've got is a person of this name." So I was able to say "Yes, that used to be me." So she said "OK, that's fine I can combine them now." And I thought that's really enlightened, she hadn't even used the name but treated me for who I am now. A little bit of thought works wonders.
>
> (Ivy, 67, trans lesbian)

This is indicative of what good practice looks like in end-of-life care; Ivy had more peace of mind once she knew that her records had been matched up and also felt reassured that this had been well handled by the staff member.

A further concern occurs for LGBT people who may live in households with more than one partner or have a number of people close to them with whom health and care professionals need to interact. This was an issue that arose for a number of participants, including a bisexual woman, Sarah. Sarah lives with two partners. She lives with a trans woman (Iris) who was previously Sarah's husband before Iris transitioned and a cis-gendered[5] man, Damian. Sarah described a period recently when she was very poorly with cancer; she had surgery and when she came home she convalesced in a room set up especially for her. She went on to explain:

> It was difficult to explain to anybody coming in why this was a change. They would come in, they would see me in that single bed in that single room, and they would see Damian and Iris, and even if they accepted that we are three, they would see they had the main bedroom, and they wouldn't realise or understand that actually normally I would have been in there too, and I would be missing it.

Celia cared for her terminally ill ex-partner Samantha, along with Samantha's ex-husband Patrick. Celia spoke about some of the health and social care professionals they encountered during this time, who made all kinds of assumptions about the relationships and/or were confused by who was who. At the same time, however, Celia felt supported by her GP and by Patrick:

> My lovely GP signed me off with stress, so that I could care for her with Patrick. And every decision was our decision, it wasn't just Patrick who was obviously her next of kin, I was consulted too.

Sarah and Celia's descriptions of networks of care are possibly, in a normative framework, quite complex to follow. Young and colleagues (1998) noted a neglect of the role of friendship and informal social networks and this is still a key area to address, where there is a range of important relationships in relation to end-of-life care. More recently, Westwood (2013) has questioned the extent to which contemporary law is adapting to take account of changing relationship forms, particularly with friendships becoming more significant in the lives of many, especially in later life and with reference to recognition of LGBT carers within key UK socio-legal policy discourses The full strength and importance of relationships which may fall under the 'umbrella' term of friendships may not be recognised. We do not yet have the language to fully encompass 'shorthand' understandings of these relationships (Almack et al., 2010) in the way that we may have some shared understandings (notwithstanding assumptions) about 'labels' such as daughter-in-law, cousin, partner, spouse and so on. Those involved in non-traditional relationships may be excluded in a number of ways, for example, not being able to have an active role in the care of the dying or by not having their grief acknowledged (Walter, 1999). These are important considerations for the investigation of the ways in which sexual orientation may impact upon concerns and experiences of end-of-life care, and on bereavement within same-sex relationships.

It is interesting to note from the above quote that although Celia felt supported in her caring role and included in decision making, it was Patrick who was noted as 'obviously' Samantha's next of kin. In the UK, this is an ambiguous term with no legal definition in terms of information sharing and decision making with/for an ill person being cared for. In practice, friends can be nominated as next of kin but this may be questioned and/or overlooked by a default position which often reverts to relationships defined by blood or filial relationships, or by marriage (although that can now of course incorporate civil partnerships and same-sex marriages). A significant number of participants had anecdotes to tell about people they knew whose family of origin had taken over when the person was dying and/or had died, leaving partners and friends without any say in decisions about their partner's or friend's care or funeral.

Some respondents in relationships had specifically taken steps to ensure that these kinds of scenarios did not arise for them:

[W]e went to some considerable length and some considerable cost to ensure that we had a level of legal protection. I mean fortunately we never really had to test that but it was reassuring for us, you know, having heard horror stories about people's partners being denied access to their bedside. So it's a little bit of protection for each other really when having to deal with each other's biological families who might potentially have a different opinion. Our civil partnership [...] that kind of gives us a whole layer of protection over and above that anyway now.

(Lydia, lesbian, 46, living with older partner)

At the time of our fieldwork, same-sex marriage had not become legal across the UK, although civil partnerships were legal in all four countries.[6] Civil partnerships were noted as an important means of 'protecting' a partner's rights to make decisions on behalf of a partner and/or to signal partners taking precedence over any members from families of origin.

A particular concern noted by two of the five trans interview participants was that, when they died, whether their family members would honour their wishes to bury them as a person of the gender with which they identify. Shirley (aged 70), who identifies as a trans woman, observed:

[T]hat's really, really important, because if [...] if it's cancelled out at the time of your demise, that just makes a mockery of your life and you as an individual.

Later in the same interview she said:

> On my demise, my daughters I'm absolutely sure would insist that I get buried as their dad, and that shouldn't be allowed, that I feel pretty strongly about. Because that's them [saying] "you're a little bit crazy, you wanted to live as a female for a while, but it's over now and you're dad again".

The Gender Recognition Act 2004 states that a person should be legally regarded as their acquired gender in all aspects of life and death. Shirley had also applied for a Gender Recognition Certificate (GRC). Despite these protections, however, she was still not confident that this would be respected on her death.

Next, we consider some of the concerns raised about the possibility of not being able to continue to live in one's home; these concerns were heightened for some by a lack of available support networks, especially for those who lived alone or who had no or few close connections with their family of origin.

Mainstream environments of care outside the home

There is some evidence to suggest that older LGBT people are often more isolated than their peer group (Stonewall, 2011) or that they are more likely to live alone. These are issues that can affect all older people due to factors such as the loss of friends and family as one ages, reduced mobility or limited income. As the UK's population ages, the issue of acute loneliness and social isolation is identified as one of the biggest challenges facing our society (Social Care Institute of Excellence, 2012). However, existing research identifies how these issues may hold particular salience for LGBT ageing populations given evidence which suggests that older LGBT people may be less likely to have any children; may be estranged from their families of origin and thus lack intergenerational support; and more likely to live alone in comparison to their heterosexual counterparts, with the incidence of living alone increasing with age (Brookdale Center on Aging, 1999; Heaphy et al., 2003). A detailed exploration of our participants' networks of support is beyond the scope of this chapter; instead we will highlight some brief considerations of accessing and using mainstream services.

In our survey, 74 per cent of respondents reported feeling 'not very confident' or 'not very confident at all' that mainstream health and social care services provide sensitive and appropriate end-of-life care services for LGBT people. The reasons why LGBT older people may lack confidence in approaching services are well documented, including the legacy of living through times of being criminalised rather than protected by law, of psychiatric interventions and other forms of prejudice and discrimination from institutions, including medicine, the church and the state.

For myself, I suppose, my fear is that, as either of us gets older or has more health problems to contend with, my fear is that not only will we have to contend with those, but we'll have to contend with the system not being very sympathetic to the fact that we're a couple.

(Ron, gay man, aged 65)

People of my sort of age who have particularly in earlier years experienced prejudicial discrimination [...] you can't predict and rely on a totally integrated service necessarily giving a feeling of safety.

(Ian, bisexual, aged 66)

It is possible that older LGBT people may delay access to health and social care services because of experiences in earlier years of discrimination and/ or fears of encountering further discrimination (Ward et al., 2010). Such anxieties mitigate against the dying person and their carers being able to have peace of mind towards the end of life and having a good experience of end-of-life care. With each new encounter with health and social care staff, LGBT people and their carers are faced with a new decision about what to disclose or hide about their sexual orientation and/or gender identity. Such decisions can be associated with concerns about whether disclosure will impact negatively upon the care they receive. Further concerns stem from negative responses from other patients, residents and clients who the older LGBT person encounters in care settings outside the home:

When my partner was dying she went to a day hospice, mainly to offer me respite. She went three times and then I was invited for the day to see what went on there. The staff introduced me as Josephine's partner to all the other patients there. The next time after when she went, no one spoke to her and they made it very, very clear why. She just wouldn't go again. She came home in tears but she wouldn't tell me why. She was a very strong independent person but obviously ill at that point. She didn't tell me about it until three days before she died. I was so emotional I didn't do anything about it then [...] but I've since taken it up with the hospice so some good might come out of it.

(Liz, lesbian, aged 65)

One time Leo was in hospital, he was distressed and said "Oh you're not going to leave me are you?" and he reached out to hold my hand [...] anyway this guy in the next bed, I could see him out the corner of my eye, sort of rear up in bed you know. After I'd gone he rang to tell the nurse, I want to move, don't want to be here. And I've never forgotten that. So, when he went in with the cancer, that was something in our minds you know, you don't make it obvious you're a gay couple. I would have loved at times to have hugged him and given him a kiss and I never felt able to.

(Ken, gay man, aged 70)

Health and social care settings don't necessarily feel like safe spaces for LGBT people to disclose important aspects about who they are and who they love, or to be able to be affectionate with their partner at a time of heightened vulnerability. Furthermore, feeling unable to access supportive provision (as in Josephine's case) or for a partner to be able to support a partner by giving them a hug (as in Ken's case) can place additional burdens on partners and friends to provide informal care, without the support of health and social care professionals.

Our data highlight many further issues to consider here in accessing mainstream services: preferences and ambivalence about the provision of LGBT specific services; experiences of discrimination (but also some positive stories about being treated with dignity and respect); decisions on an ongoing basis about whether or not to disclose information about their sexual orientation, and strategies to keep such information hidden. Even those who have been open about their sexual orientation in the past may find that they are less confident in doing so if they become frail or need more support from a wider range of people.

A key finding in our data was that forms of discrimination are not always overt but may include more subtle and sometimes unintentional forms of discrimination that are less easy to challenge. One example is 'heteronormativity', a cultural bias that views heterosexuality as 'normal' and taken for granted in a way that LGBT relationships and identities are not. Examples of heteronormativity include the under-representation of LGBT relationships and people in service promotion leaflets, or assumptions made that someone is heterosexual unless otherwise stated. Heteronormativity can make someone feel invisible, erase a big part of someone's identity, and impact upon their ability to involve those closest to them in their care. Some examples we were told by interview respondents include a bisexual woman sat in the waiting room with her female partner; when the nurse called her in she said: "Your sister can come with you." In contrast, if it was a man and woman sat together of similar age, it is more likely that the nurse might check (or assume) first that they are husband and wife and not brother and sister. Questions about children and grandchildren may appear friendly attempts at conversation, but for many older LGBT people having children wasn't a possibility or they might be estranged. This 'pervasive experience of heterosexism' (Cox, 2011, p. 194) can render a central aspect of one's identity as invisible. Service providers frequently either do not consider that some service recipients may be LGBT and/or suggest that they provide inclusive services by treating everyone the same (see e.g. GRAI (GLBTI Retirement Association Inc), 2010).

Conclusions

To be living with a life-limiting condition, to be dying or bereaved can be socially excluding experiences and there are additional layers of exclusion that LGBT people may face at these times. This may include feeling unable to disclose their sexual orientation or their gender identity or other aspects of their lifestyle and culture due to previous experiences or concerns about discrimination from wider society (and sometimes for bisexual people, discrimination from within L&G communities). As a LGB or T person, making decisions about what to say and to whom about your sexual orientation or gender identity is constant and can be very wearing, especially if you are already feeling ill or vulnerable.

If LGBT people are not confident about services or staff, they may not seek support and/or may not feel able to speak about matters and people who are important to them and crucial to dying well. It is often said about end-of-life care that we only have one chance to get it right. In caring for or providing services for LGBT people at the end of life this also takes on an additional meaning. LGBT people may have experienced encounters with health and social care staff at some point in their lives where they feel unacknowledged, invisible or in some other way excluded – often against a background of a lifetime of such instances. LGBT people will be adept and alert to nuanced responses upon disclosing information about their sexual orientation or gender identity. Every encounter with someone new can be accompanied by concerns about how that individual will respond to information about a LGBT identity. Any points of disclosure can be critical one-chance moments – if not met positively this can be a missed opportunity to build up caring relationships and to get to know the whole person which is central to holistic end-of-life care. However, if LGBT people and those close to them do need care or other services, it is so important that they are able to feel safe in approaching services for assistance and that services are prepared to encounter LGBT people, such that it becomes an embedded part of service provision towards and at the end of life.

Notes

1 Acknowledgments and thanks to the Research Fellows who worked with me on this project – Anne Patterson and Meiko Makita. Thanks also go to the project co-applicants and advisory group and of course to all the participants who generously gave their time to this research.
2 Estimating the size and demographic trends of the ageing LGBT population is difficult. The UK Department of Trade and Industry (DTI, 2003) cites an estimate of 5 to 7 per cent nationally. To date in the UK, the Census has not included specific questions about people's sexual orientation/gender identity. Difficulties in collecting such data requiring self-identification are also more complex than simply asking the questions; some people may not want to disclose that information or not want to identify with the categories provided.
3 The UK ranks first in the 2015 Quality of Death Index, a measure of the quality of palliative care in 80 countries around the world (report by The Economist Intelligence Unit).
4 Pathways to LGBT identities; factors impacting upon coming out or transitioning; accessibility to help and support at current age; talking about ageing; advance planning for future and end-of-life care; religion or spirituality; experiences within health and social care settings (for oneself or as a carer); preferences for how services should be organised.
5 Cisgender is a term for people whose gender identity matches the sex that they were assigned at birth.

6 It is now possible for same-sex couples to get married in England and Wales (from 29 March 2014) and in Scotland (from December 2014) or to convert a civil partnership into a marriage in England, Scotland and Wales. Civil partnerships are legal in Northern Ireland but not same-sex marriage.

References

Almack, K. (2016) 'Dying, death and bereavement', in Goldberg, AE. (ed.), *The SAGE Encyclopaedia of LGBTQ Studies*. New York: Sage, pp. 342–347.

Almack, K., Seymour, J. and Bellamy, G. (2010) 'Exploring the impact of sexual orientation on experiences and concerns about end of life care and on bereavement for lesbian, gay and bisexual elders', *Sociology*, 44(5): 908–924.

Bristowe, K., Hodson, M., Wee, B., Almack, K., Johnson, K., Daveson, BA., Koffman, J., McEnhill, L. and Harding, R. (2018) 'Recommendations to reduce inequalities for LGBT people facing advanced illness: ACCESSCare national qualitative interview study', *Palliative Medicine*, 32: 23–35.

Brookdale Center on Aging (1999) *Assistive Housing for Elderly Gays and Lesbians in New York City*, New York: Hunter College and Senior Action in a Gay Environment (SAGE).

Brotman, S., Ryan, B., Collins, S., Chamberland, L., Cormier, R., Julien, D., Meyer, E., Peterkin, A. and Richard, B. (2007) 'Coming out to care: Caregivers of gay and lesbian seniors in Canada', *The Gerontologist*, 47(4): 490–503.

Cartwright, C., Hughes, M. and Lienert, T. (2012) 'End-of-life care for gay, lesbian, bisexual and transgender people', *Culture, Health & Sexuality*, 14(5): 537–548.

Cox, K (2011) 'Sexual orientation', in Oliviere, D., Monroe, B. and Payne, S. (eds), *Death, Dying and Social Difference* (2nd edn). Oxford: Oxford University Press, pp. 191–199.

CQC (2016) *A Different Ending: Addressing inequalities in end of life care (Overview Report)*. London: Care Quality Commission.

Department of Health (DoH) (2008a) *End of Life Care Strategy: Promoting high quality care for all adults at the end of life*. London: Department of Health.

Department of Health (DoH) (2008b) *The End of Life Care Strategy: Promoting high quality care for all adults at the end of life. Equality Impact Assessment*. London: Department of Health.

Department of Trade and Industry (DTI) (2003) *Civil Partnership: A framework for the legal recognition of same-sex couples*, London: DTI Women and Equality Unit: 68.

Gomes, B. and Higginson, IJ. (2008) 'Where people die (1974–2030): Past trends, future projections and implications for care', *Palliative Medicine*, 22(1): 33–41.

GRAI (GLBTI Retirement Association Inc) (2010) *"We Don't Have Any of Those People Here": Retirement accommodation and aged care issues for non-heterosexual populations*. Western Australia: GRAI.

Hall, S., Petkova, H., Tsouros, AD., Costantini, M. and Higginson, IJ. (2011) *Palliative Care for Older People: Better practices*. Denmark: WHO Regional Office for Europe.

Harding, R., Epiphaniou, E. and Chidgey-Clark, J. (2012) 'Needs, experiences, and preferences of sexual minorities for end-of-life care and palliative care: A systematic review', *Journal of Palliative Medicine*, 15(5): 602–611.

Heaphy, B., Yip, AKT. and Thompson, D. (2003) *Lesbian, Gay and Bisexual Lives Over 50.* Nottingham: York House Publications.

Kennedy, S., Seymour, J., Almack, K. and Cox, K. (2009) 'Key stakeholders' experiences and views of the NHS End of Life Care Programme: Findings from a national evaluation', *Palliative Medicine*, 23(4): 283–294.

Lawton, A., White, J. and Fromme, EK. (2013) 'End-of-life and advance care planning considerations for lesbian, gay, bisexual, and transgender patients #275', *Journal of Palliative Medicine*, 17(1): 106–108.

Leadbeater, C. and Garber, J. (2010) *Dying for Change.* London: DEMOS.

Manthorpe, J. (2003) 'Nearest and dearest? The neglect of lesbians in caring relationships', *British Journal of Social Work*, 33(6): 753–768.

NHS England (2014) *NHS England's Actions for End of Life Care.* Leeds: NHS England.

ONS (2015) *Mid-2014 Population Estimates UK.* London: Office for National Statistics.

Plummer, K. (2007) 'The call of life stories in ethnographic research', in Atkinson, PE, Coffey, A., Delamont, S., Lofland, J. and Lofland, L. (eds), *The Handbook of Ethnography.* London: Sage, pp. 395–406.

Pollock, K. (2015) 'Is home always the best and preferred place of death?', *BMJ*, 10 October, pp. 18–19.

Price, E. (2010) 'Coming out to care: Gay and lesbian carers' experiences of dementia services', *Health & Social Care in the Community*, 18(2): 160–168.

Rawlings, D. (2012) 'End-of-life care considerations for gay, lesbian, bisexual, and transgender individuals', *International Journal of Palliative Nursing*, 18(1): 29–34.

Ruth, K. and Verne, J. (2010) *Deaths in Older Adults in England.* Bristol: National End of Life Care Intelligence Network.

Saunders, C. (1976) 'Care of the dying: The problem of euthanasia', *Nursing Times*, 72(27): 1049–1051.

Social Care Institute of Excellence (2012) *Preventing Loneliness and Social Isolation among Older People. At a glance briefing.* London: SCIE.

Stonewall (2011) *Lesbian, Gay and Bisexual People in Later Life.* London: Stonewall.

Victor, CR. (2010) *Ageing, Health and Care.* Bristol: Policy Press.

Walter, T. (1999) *On Bereavement.* Buckingham: Open University Press.

Ward, R., Pugh, S. and Price, E. (2010) *Don't Look Back? Improving health and social care service delivery for older LGB users.* Manchester: Equality and Human Rights Commission.

Westwood, S. (2013) '"My friends are my family": An argument about the limitations of contemporary law's recognition of relationships in later life', *Journal of Social Welfare and Family Law*, 35(3): 347–363.

Wilkinson, R. and Marmot, M. (2003) *Social Determinants of Health: The solid facts* (2nd edn). Denmark: WHO Regional Office for Europe.

Young, E., Seale, C. and Bury, M. (1998) '"It's not like family going is it?" Negotiating friendship boundaries towards the end of life', *Mortality*, 3(1): 27–42.

12 Not 'just a nice thing to do'

The effects of austerity on LGBT older people

Martin Mitchell, Mehul Kotecha and Malen Davies

Introduction

This chapter presents the findings of qualitative research conducted by NatCen[1] Social Research on behalf of the public services trade union UNISON[2] (Mitchell et al., 2013; Davies et al., 2016). The aim of the study was to examine whether austerity was affecting the lives of lesbian, gay, bisexual and transgender (LGBT) people and the services they used, and, if so, in what ways? The study was first conducted in 2013 and repeated in 2016 to achieve further depth of insight into these issues and to see what had changed in services for LGBT once austerity had been in place for a longer time.

Although the study was focused on LGBT people in general, and on people providing services to LGBT people, LGBT people from older age groups participated in both the 2013 and 2016 studies. Consequently, the findings were re-examined to see whether there were specific issues of concern to older LGBT people. In line with the *English Longitudinal Study of Ageing*[3] we took older people to be 50-plus years old, although the way in which we categorised age for both waves of the study means that some people who were in the 46 to 56 age group (namely 46 to 49 years old) have been included because it was not possible to separate them out.

The overall finding from this re-analysis was that, while not all LGBT older people were affected by public sector spending cuts, there were a number of ways in which they were. Participants who were affected described experiences which appeared to suggest that a reduction in funding for specialist services and supports for LGBT older people made some of them feel isolated and marginalised. In particular, there was a picture of distinctive needs among LGBT older people being treated as 'a nice thing to do' which could no longer be afforded in times of austerity. This was without adequate alternative mainstream services and appropriate training for staff in those services being put in place.

In this chapter, the experiences of our participants are described in the context of reductions in public sector spending. This is then followed by combined findings from the 2013 and 2016 studies. We first look at reasons why some LGBT people said they were not affected by the cuts. We then go on to explore the findings in relation to four areas of important issues emerging from the data. These were (1) worsening pay and conditions; (2) loss of specialist LGBT services and service providers; (3) a sense of growing isolation and lack of social support; and (4) the marginalisation of specific LGBT people's needs in policy and service provision.

Context

'Austerity' and cuts in public expenditure

In May 2010, the UK Conservative–Liberal Democrat Coalition government began introducing a series of significant and sustained reductions in public spending intended to reduce the budget deficit. Often referred to as *austerity cuts,* these reductions have continued since 2015 under the current Conservative government and entail cuts in funding to or via government departments and in local authorities. Exceptions to the cuts were front-line spending in the National Health Service, non-investment funding in schools, and spending on international development, which were largely ring-fenced and protected (Crawford et al., 2013). The devolved governments were also expected to receive significant cuts in their block grants between 2010 and 2016.

The Institute of Fiscal Studies (IFS, 2015) estimated that the magnitude of cuts felt by non-protected government departments would be 20.6 per cent on average in 2016.[4] The 2016 budget announced a further intended £3.5 billion savings across non-protected departments by 2019/2020. It is unclear at this stage how the extent of austerity may be affected by the UK referendum decision to leave the European Union or by the Conservative Party's failure to win a government majority in the 2017 general election. Other cuts and their effects have occurred through job freezes, changes to pensions and 1 per cent pay caps in the public sector. They have also occurred through contracting out of public services to the voluntary sector and the competitive tendering for services in that sector, which sometimes reduced wages and staffing levels in those services.

Although the austerity cuts impact upon the UK as a whole, cuts in local authority (LA) spending and their associated service providers have meant that some areas, organisations and groups are disproportionately affected, particularly the most vulnerable. For instance, a recent report by the Joseph Rowntree Foundation (Hastings et al., 2015) suggests that more deprived local authorities experienced greater cuts compared to more affluent ones, contributing to rising inequalities between different local authority areas and the communities they serve. It has been argued that austerity cuts have specific significance for LGBT people because many of the specialist services provided to them are either directly provided by local authorities or are commissioned by them in the voluntary sector (Public and Commercial Services Union, 2012; Colgan et al., 2014).

The effects of austerity measures should also be seen within the context of a reported high level of demand for LGBT services. This arises due to continuing discrimination still faced by LGBT people in the UK, despite the introduction of the Equality Act 2010, and a consequent need for specialist services (Colgan et al., 2014). Reduction in funding for services to LGBT people can therefore have effects on service users, the specialists delivering those services, and on the quality and responsiveness of services remaining after cuts in funding have been made.

Policy changes in funding a delivery of services

Specific challenges of austerity on small and medium-sized LGBT charities exacerbate the impact of cuts upon LGBT populations. With reference to such organisations, a recent evidence review by the Institute of Public Policy Research (IPPR) (Hunter et al., 2016) found that smaller and medium-sized charities – which are often providers of services for LGBT people – were disproportionately affected by cuts in public funding. A recent example of this is the closure of the Project for Advocacy, Counselling and Education (PACE) in 2016,[5] a smaller London-based charity which has provided counselling and advice services since 1985 (Public and Commercial Services Union, 2012). The IPPR also reported that small and medium-sized charities have been particularly affected by a move towards funding patterns which favour contract (over grants) and a competitive model of commissioning in which providers of all sizes and types compete to deliver public services. This sometimes led to larger, more mainstream organisations dominating provision, and the needs of LGBT people having to compete for space and time in services targeted at wider equality and discrimination concerns.

Mainstreaming of sexual orientation and gender identity in policy and service delivery

Another influence on the reduction in funding for LGBT services is the idea that they should be provided as part of mainstream services such as health and social care. In many cases the drive towards so called 'mainstreaming' of equality concerns is based on a genuine desire to make all services more inclusive for everyone (McNaughton-Nicholls et al., 2010). In relation to research on the Public Sector Equality Duty[6] (PSED), however, there were instances when attempts were made to try to mainstream services before staff had a full understanding of the needs of specific groups they were supposed to serve (Arthur et al., 2013). The coincidence of attempts to mainstream equalities with austerity sometimes appeared to have been used to cut funding to specialist LGBT services. Yet, the way in which this affected the recipients of those services is not properly understood.

Despite the significance of austerity cuts to the LGBT community, there is a paucity of evidence on whether this has impacted upon LGBT populations. Colgan et al.'s (2014) study of the impact of austerity cuts upon the LGBT voluntary and community sector (VCS) is a notable exception, but even in this study the focus is primarily on the experience and views of service providers. Considering this gap in knowledge, NatCen were commissioned by UNISON in 2013 to explore perceptions of whether and how austerity measures have affected LGBT people as service providers *and* users in the UK. The study was repeated in 2016 to provide an update on the original research (Davies et al., 2016).

Methodology

Methods

In 2013 UNISON commissioned NatCen to conduct a small-scale study into the experiences of LGBT people, and the people providing services to them, in the context of austerity. Both waves of the research in 2013 and 2016 were qualitative and used two data-collection methods: (1) written submissions in response to open questions via a secure website; (2) in-depth interviews to explore a range of purposively selected issues and experiences within the LGBT populations.

Written submission consisted of participants providing responses to six key open-ended questions:

- Whether services have been affected and in what ways.
- Whether cuts have affected individuals, including LGBT people, their friends, families, colleagues and the wider LGBT community.
- Examples of effects on LGBT individuals.
- Examples of effects on income and expenditure of LGBT individuals.
- Suggestions for ways to respond to cuts.
- Any other comments.

The same questions were asked again in 2016. The nature of written submissions varied considerably, from short comments to much lengthier written contributions.

The in-depth interviews involved purposively selecting participants for telephone interviews from those who had completed an online submission and/or agreed to take part in the interview. Selection was based on achieving diversity across a number of criteria, including their relationship to service use and provision (i.e. service user, provider or both), their UNISON membership (whether they were a member or not), their gender, sexual orientation, gender identity (transgender) and age. Telephone interviews lasted between 30 minutes to an hour and were conducted using a topic guide covering such themes as:

- Whether and how austerity had affected LGBT service users and providers.
- Responses to cuts as a LGBT person, service provider or in another capacity.
- Key messages about the research topic.

Written submissions were collected directly via a secure website. Interviews were digitally recorded and the data organised thematically and analysed alongside written submission using the *Framework* approach (Ritchie et al., 2013).

Recruitment

In the 2013 study participants were recruited via UNISON's LGBT network and other contacts known to UNISON (e.g. trans members' networks). UNISON sent an email to all relevant individuals on behalf of NatCen. The email contained information about the study and a link to a secure website that provided further information about the study and where participants could make a written submission, make a submission and volunteer to take part in a follow-up in-depth interview, or simply volunteer to be interviewed. UNISON members were invited to pass information about the study on to others to whom the research would be relevant.

In 2016, the same procedure was followed except for broadening recruitment through a range of LGBT organisations and other organisations providing services to LGBT people. One aim of the 2016 study was to move deliberately beyond primary reliance on UNISON members and their contacts to broaden the data collected.

Achieved samples

In 2013, 101 participants took part in the study (89 made written submissions only; 9 made written submissions and were followed up because they offered specific insights; and 3 took part in interviews only where they were unable to participate online). Twenty-five were in older age groups, including 14 aged 46 to 55 and 11 aged 56 to 65). A good diversity was achieved across all participants in terms of gender, sexual orientation and gender identity.

In 2016, 183 people took part in the study. We received 176 written submissions from participants, 11 of whom also took part in a follow-up in-depth interview; an additional 7 people took part in an in-depth interview only. In the 2016 study 83 were aged 46 or over, which was a higher proportion of

Table 12.1 Achieved sample by older age groups and sexual orientation in the 2016 study

Age group	Gay or lesbian	Bisexual	Heterosexual*	Other**	Prefer not to say	Total
46–55	37	7	4	3	2	53
56–65	14	3	3	2	1	23
66–75	4	-	1	2	-	7
Total	55	10	8	7	3	83

Notes
* e.g. a service provider offering services to LGBT people.
** Most people who responded in this way answered as transgender, possibly as a result of the question on sexual orientation appearing before the questions on gender identity during collection of demographic information.

Table 12.2 Achieved sample by older age groups and gender identity in response to the question: 'Have you gone through any part of a process (including thoughts or actions) to change from the sex you were described as at birth to the gender you identify with, or do you intend to?

Age group	Yes (transgender)	No (cisgender)	Prefer not to say	Total
46–55	9	43	1	**53**
56–65	10	13	-	**13**
66–75	2	5	-	**7**
Total	**21**	**61**	**1**	**83**

LGBT older participants than in the 2013 study. A breakdown of older participants by age, sexual orientation and gender identity is shown in Tables 12.1 and 12.2.

Limitations of the study

The study was based on participants' self-reported perceptions of cuts to services, including both service providers and users. It should be noted that it was not always easy to attribute the observed reductions in funding and services directly to austerity measures, and to disentangle the effects of austerity measures from effects of persistent homophobia, biphobia and transphobia and discrimination towards the LGBT community. The use of qualitative data also means that we cannot draw conclusions about the prevalence of different views, nor make a wider assessment of the impact of austerity measures. Instead, the focus is on mapping the range of different types of cuts and their effects. To this extent the study provides insights into the nature and effects of austerity on some LGBT older people but does not claim that all LGBT older people are affected in the ways described. Most data in the study also related to lesbians and gay men. Further research is needed on issues specifically affecting people who identify as bisexual and transgender.

Findings

Not affected

Not all people who took part in the study said they were affected by austerity cuts. Some commentators have tried to account for the fact that although the scale of cuts has been significant, they have not been felt by most of the population. In an opinion poll *Ipsos Mori* found that, in 2013, 48 per cent of the public agreed with the statement that 'budget cuts have gone too far and threaten social unrest'; by contrast 65 per cent said they had not noticed a change in the quality of local services personally and, in some cases, satisfaction with local authority services had gone up.

Part of the explanation for these findings may be that the public sector is less efficient when it has more money to spend and that public sector workers have devised ways to deliver services more efficiently so that they can be protected. Another argument, however, is that the effect of cuts is concentrated on sections of the population that are most vulnerable and least likely to complain (in this sense general population surveys may not be the best indicator of austerity effects) (Flanders, 2013).

The extent to which people were affected by the reductions in public sector funding in these studies varied. Some older LGBT said they were 'not affected' at all. The main reasons why LGBT people said they had not experienced cuts were: (1) there were few or no LGBT services in their area to be cut; (2) that the services they used (such as health services) had been protected from spending cuts to date; (3) they had no awareness of cuts personally due to lack of information; (4) they thought cuts only affected the most disadvantaged and vulnerable; (5) services had been restructured to make them more efficient and to protect service users from cuts for the time being. Some participants also said that, while they were not personally affected, their partners or others they knew had been.

It is important not to dismiss the views and experiences of participants who were unaffected by cuts in public services. Yet, at the same time, there are two reasons for concentrating on those who were affected. First, as a qualitative study the emphasis was to represent the range and diversity of experiences within the sample population. Second, because, even if only a relatively small number of participants were affected by public spending cuts, their experiences are important in being able to show where service users are most affected and/or where services were failing. This section of the chapter draws out the ways in which older LGBT people said they were affected by reductions in public spending.

As discussed above, we found from our sample that four themes emerged in terms of the ways in which older LGBT people were affected. These were:

- Worsening pay and conditions (following a similar pattern with other age groups).
- Loss of specialist LGBT services and service providers.
- A sense of growing isolation and lack of social support.
- The marginalisation of specific LGBT needs.

Given that LGBT older people were not the specific focus of either study, it is unlikely that these themes will be exhaustive. Further research is needed to explore these and other potential factors affecting LGBT older people further.

Worsening pay and conditions

In some instances, concerns arising from austerity were the same for older LGBT people as they were for all LGBT people who took part in the research. This was particularly the case in relation to concerns about pay and conditions arising from public sector cuts. A recurring message from LGBT people, for themselves and for those who they knew in the wider LGBT community, was the actual or anticipated financial hardship caused by the cuts. Some participants expressed strong anxiety over reductions in their incomes arising from redundancies, below-inflation pay rises and from benefit cuts.

Among the participants who expressed concerns about and/or who experienced financial hardships there were a range of concerns. In relation to employment, shifts in employment patterns to zero-hour contracts, and people being moved from stable work to roll-over short-term contracts by their employer were of concern to some in terms of current earnings and financial security. Other LGBT people worried about their longer term future financial security; for example, their inability to save towards major items like a house, their future job prospects and pensions.

Concerns were especially expressed by participants working in the public sector or in services that had been contracted out from the public sector to the voluntary sector. For example, in one case an older transgender participant commented on the way in which a pay freeze and re-grading had affected her:

> Due to working in local government, I have not had a pay rise in three years, despite earning under £21,000. Plus, my job has been re-graded and I now earn less money.
>
> (Trans woman, service provider, 46 to 55 age group,
> UNISON member, 2013)

Such pay freezes were described as having real effects for some older LGBT people. For instance, in one case a participant said she was left out of pocket due to budget cuts by their employer, and with another older LGBT community worker having to fund her own travel expenses. One older lesbian working in a public sector mental health service said:

> I'm forced to make reductions in purchases like social, groceries, heating bills because of reduced income.
>
> (Lesbian, service provider, 56 to 65 age group,
> not a UNISON member, 2013)

Our sample included both the views of managers and front-line staff delivering services. From the management point of view some providers said that they had tried to restructure or remodel their services to be more efficient and to protect service users as far as possible from the worst of austerity cuts' effects. However, even those who held this view recognised that 'weathering' such cuts usually created greater workloads for staff in the medium to long term until further funding could be found. From the view of front-line providers, restructuring or remodelling was often experienced, not only as increases in demand for services but also as worse pay and worse terms and conditions.

> Where the services are commissioned out it is noticeable how pay has fallen and jobs are usually on short-term contracts.
>
> (Lesbian, service provider, 46 to 55 age group,
> UNISON member, 2016)

There is evidence that LGBT people are more likely to work in the public and voluntary sectors because they feel they will receive less discrimination there (Mitchell et al., 2009 section 6.2). Worse pay and conditions in this respect may have a double impact upon LGBT people. On the one hand, they might be disproportionately affected by pay freezes in the sector; on the other, they will be older LGBT people in receipt of those services.

Loss of LGBT specialist services and service providers

'Catch all' services

A theme found among older service providers and service users was that LGBT specialist services and service providers were being lost owing to reductions in public sector funding. Yet, at the same time, more mainstream services were not thought to be responding adequately to the needs of LGBT service users, including older LGBT people. One aspect of this was that the service providers of LGBT services related to mental health, counselling, domestic abuse and safer sex were being asked by commissioners of services to broaden their remit to survive. As one service provider put it, they thought they were being asked to be 'catch all' services:

> We are being asked to be all in one, singing and dancing diversity organisation. We specialise in the LGBT, [populations and] we can understand race, disability and religion as we will have people in the organisation who can help with this but it's not our focus. [...] we aren't going to be experts in this field.
>
> (Lesbian, service user and provider, 46 to 55 age group, not a UNISON member, 2016)

This theme was also reflected in the way in which more mainstream services were expected to take on the role of provision that might previously have been provided or complemented by LGBT specific services, whether in the public or voluntary sector. An important point made in this respect by one older service user was that public sector commissioners were sometimes not commissioning LGBT services, even when they did not have sufficient data to decide whether such services were needed or not. She thought that if commissioners and services were not collecting data on their users' sexuality (sexual orientation) they would not be able to meet their service users' needs.

> I am aware that mental health services – some of which are within the NHS – are not all recording sexuality on their demographics; and if they are recording it they are not looking at the data to see if their services are reaching the LGBT community.
>
> (Lesbian, service user, 56 to 65 age group, not a UNISON member, 2016)

This perspective was demonstrated more clearly by an older transgender service user who experienced mental health issues but who felt increasingly unable to find the specialist advice she needed.

> As a trans person I often experience bouts of depression and anxiety, whilst I can still function in day-to-day life having the outlet to talk through these is important. Such [advice and support] services are much harder to find.
>
> (Trans woman, service user, 46 to 55 age group, UNISON member, 2016)

Public sector service providers and commissioners will therefore need to be clearer about the extent and nature of LGBT older people's needs and whether they can be satisfied within broader services.

Loss of older LGBT specialist service providers

One effect of reduced funding for services was thought to be that valuable staff with specialist knowledge were lost as they were made redundant or their role was taken over by someone with a wider remit. This same theme re-emerged in the 2016 study, with a service provider emphasising that a key effect of austerity cuts was:

> A reduction in the quality of support given. [...] The service list staff who had years of experience in the sector, the opportunity to share expertise with partner orgs is reduced.
>
> (Lesbian, service provider and user, 46 to 55 age group, not a UNISON member, 2016)

The loss of longer serving, older LGBT specialists was regarded as having negative effects on services and their service users. Some examples of the effects highlighted in the research from both 2013 and 2016 included: (1) the loss of networks and information sharing between experienced staff with their network; (2) an increase in the knowledge gap of the workforce who support LGBT people; (3) fewer experienced staff available to provide services leading to less people having access to the right kind of support. Participants in the 2013 study thought that services would be less likely to be able to respond appropriately and quickly to a person's needs and that services could be delivered in discriminatory ways. The consequences for older LGBT workers were less clear and require further investigation.

Isolation and lack of social support

One effect of the perceived greater invisibility and marginalisation of LGBT people was that some older LGBT people said they felt more isolated and less connected with a LGBT community than in the past. The loss of and reduction in service provision and opportunities to meet away from the pubs, clubs and apps of the gay scene was key to this growing sense of isolation. This was because it provided important 'non-scene' support for older LGBT people, especially those without support from their family.

> [I] don't feel as connected to the community; have lost network of support; more isolated because they're not as available.
>
> (Gay man, service provider and user, 56 to 65 age group, not a UNISON member, 2013)

There are no publicly funded local places to meet away from the gay scene. I don't really like the way older gay men are treated in pubs and clubs but there isn't much alternative where I live.

> (Gay man, service user, 56 to 65 age group,
> not a UNISON member, 2016)

The closure of or reduction in the following services and opportunities for meeting other LGBT people particularly heightened a sense of isolation for some older LGBT people. Reported loss or reduction of funding and services included:

- Peer support from other LGBT people, for example, in day centres.
- LGBT centres offering advice and support and a safe place for LGBT people to meet (e.g. left in limbo when a council-funded LGBT support group and outreach project reduced the services it provided).
- Fewer LGBT events, such as Pride events, taking place in local, non-commercial settings.

The impact of the reduction and closure of these services was vividly expressed by a service user in terms of:

> [There are] less options to meet other older LGBT people and share worries and information. No longer can meet at day centres. Support activities of local LGBT advice centre severely curtailed.
>
> (Gay man, service user, 66 to 75 age group,
> not a UNISON member, 2016)

These issues tended to be more evident in the accounts of older gay men; a tendency which was also shown through research on the *Opening Doors*[7] project which identified that more gay men than lesbians were dependent on this member organisation's non-scene social activities and support (Knocker et al., 2012).

Mental health service users and providers also thought that LGBT people would be more anxious, frustrated and concerned because of cuts to services that would otherwise have supported them. Some participants thought that their sense of well-being might decline because of growing feelings of isolation and greater feelings of financial insecurity. This impact was captured in the experiences of one older lesbian who had used domestic violence and HIV support services.

> HIV and domestic violence services cut or reduced [...] [which] affected my self-esteem and coping mechanism.
>
> (Lesbian, service user, 46 to 55 age group,
> not a UNISON member, 2016)

Indeed, another participant in the 2016 service referred specifically to closure of the *Broken Rainbow*[8] service – which provided support related to domestic violence in same sex couples – as a cut that had affected them directly. Similar closures were also reported by other participants:

> The local LGBT counselling service closed down so [it is] difficult to access LGBT focused counselling if I or my clients need one.
>
> (Lesbian, service provider and user, 46 to 55 age group, 2016)

As a result of these types of spending reductions and cuts, participants felt that LGBT people were not receiving the same quality of support and/ or medical treatment as they had in the past and that this was affecting their mental health. Poorer quality mental health services included reduced availability of appointments, early discharge from services, lack of relevant services or staff such as counsellors trained in issues facing LGBT people, and cutting essential services such as help lines. Feelings of a lack of support away from the LGBT scene, and a lack of places to meet and share worries with others, were therefore two ways in which older LGBT people seemed to be especially placed at a disadvantage by austerity cuts.

Marginalisation, invisibility and guilt

The final theme to emerge among older LGBT participants was that austerity and reductions in public sector spending meant that specialist services targeted at LGBT people were seen as less important by service commissioners in times of scare resources. There were two dimensions to these views.

The first was that there was pressure to merge LGBT concerns with other wider equality and diversity concerns in trying to challenge discrimination and promote equality. The concern which participants expressed was that issues faced by LGBT people tended to be seen as less important than other disadvantaged groups. As a consequence, LGBT people became marginalised and more invisible, with the issues they faced specifically being 'lost' among a range of other issues. An example of this was a LGBT advisory forum on public services supported by a local authority. As the participant put it:

> There are pressures for the LGB and T network to become part of a wider advisory forum. We feel that LGBT issues have tended to get lost in that forum [...] one person said to me, "to be honest I stopped going because I didn't feel there was enough focus on LGBT issues."
>
> (Gay man, service user, 45 to 56 age group, not a UNISON member, 2013)

The closing of or reduced offers from LGBT services also had the added effect of reducing the visibility of LGBT people. An older lesbian participant articulated this feeling clearly in terms of LGBT people being 'out of sight' and easily removed from the policy agenda in times of austerity:

> LGBT issues are traditionally out of sight and easily removed or placed in a 'nice to do if we could afford it, never, never' category and this only increases in times of austerity.
>
> (Lesbian, service user, 56 to 65 age group,
> UNISON member, 2013)

She therefore felt a sense that LGBT issues or services were not being prioritised.

A second dimension was that, as a result of being deprioritised, service providers were sometimes regarded as becoming desensitised to the experiences of LGBT needs and that LGBT people might not receive an appropriate service. For instance, one older lesbian service user described the way in which she felt a GP had asked inappropriate questions during a consultation, despite treating her and her partners as lesbians separately. In this instance, the participant felt that the reason she was not treated correctly was because her GP was not as knowledgeable about her needs as a more specialist LGBT service provider might be.

Others, however, put such treatment in the wider context of cuts in services, training and resources, which meant that service providers simply had less time to deal with the individual needs of their service users. For instances, a gay male service user and provider said:

> Providing welcoming and person-centred services means an investment in time and training for staff. Training opportunities are less available due to cuts, staff feel pressured to do as little as necessary to help customers, they won't go the extra mile for customers because management don't value it […] all of which makes the customer experience less satisfactory.
>
> (Gay man, service user and provider, 46 to 55 age group,
> UNISON member, 2016)

Underpinning such feelings of inappropriate treatment and marginalisation was the view that sometimes LGBT people were treated by policy makers and service providers as problematic because their needs differed from the *norm* in times of scarce resources. This raised questions about whether funders, commissioners and service providers do see services for LGBT people as simply a 'nice thing to do' or, as this participant put it:

> like wanting LGBT groups or adults is somewhat of a luxury at work when there are so many other pressing demands.
>
> (Lesbian, service user, 46 to 55 age group,
> UNISON member, 2013)

Clearly, resources may need to be rationalised in times of public spending reductions. It should be asked, however, whether it is too easy to cut services to LGBT older people because of the perceived small size of the community by some commissioners. The relative invisibility of LGBT people compared to other minority or disadvantaged groups also arguably makes them more vulnerable to cuts. This research suggests that specialist services for LGBT are not simply a 'nice thing to do' for some older LGBT people. Such services are in many instances essential to ensure that services feel inclusive to LGBT and LGBT older people.

Conclusions

This study provides initial insights into the way in which some older LGBT people are experiencing the effects of austerity as reductions in public spending that have been happening over the past few years. While some participants were not experiencing any effects, this did not mean that others were not vulnerable to them.

Older LGBT people told us that – like other people of working age – some of them were experiencing worsening pay and conditions, especially as services to LGBT people moved from the public to the voluntary sector and smaller charities received cuts in their public funding.

The closure of specialist LGBT services (such as PACE and Broken Rainbow) was a concern in circumstances where participants felt that mainstream services were not adequately sensitive to their needs. The disappearance of such services – which also acted as 'non-scene' places for LGBT people to meet, share worries and gain support – was also of particular concern to older LGBT people, especially gay men. This sometimes led to a sense of social isolation, lack of support and the possibility of declining mental health for a group of LGBT older people.

The findings suggest that the needs of some LGBT people were being marginalised or being mainstreamed in broader service delivery models in circumstances where they were de-prioritised or not fully understood. Indeed, a recurring theme was that LGBT people believed their needs were regarded as a 'luxury' rather than as important issues with specific consequences for their lives. Service providers and commissioners will find it useful to examine the themes raised in this research in order to find out whether they are responding to the needs of older LGBT people appropriately when organising their services. In specific circumstances, providing services for older LGBT people will not just be a 'nice thing to do' but essential to provide appropriate care and support.

Notes

1 NatCen Social Research (formerly the National Centre for Social Research) is the UK's largest independent, non-politically aligned and not-for-profit social research organisation: www.natcen.ac.uk/.

2 UNISON is one of Britain largest unions, serving 1.3 million members providing services in the public and private sectors: www.unison.org.uk/about/.
3 The English Longitudinal Study of Ageing (ELSA) is a unique and rich resource of information on the health, social, well-being and economic circumstances of the English population aged 50 and older: www.elsa-project.ac.uk/.
4 This government has delivered substantial spending cuts; big differences in parties' plans for next parliament. Available at http://election2015.ifs.org.uk/public-spending (accessed 20 July 2016).
5 Reference to the closure of PACE: https://londonqueers.wordpress.com/2016/01/30/what-does-the-closure-of-pace-mean-for-londons-lgbtq-communities/.
6 The PSED is the part of the Equality Act (2010) which places a duty of public sector bodies and organisations they fund to eliminate unlawful discrimination, promote equality of opportunity and foster good relations between groups sharing a protected characteristic.
7 Opening Doors is a membership organisation providing regular social activities and which aims to develop local networks for LGBT people 50 and over (e.g. Opening Doors London: http://openingdoorslondon.org.uk/).
8 see Mitchell et al. (2013, p. 16): http://natcen.ac.uk/media/205545/unison-lgbt-austerity-final-report.pdf.

References

Arthur, S., Mitchell, M., Graham, J. and Beninger, K. (2013) *Views and Experiences of the Public Sector Equality Duty (PSED): Qualitative research to inform the review.* London: Government Equalities Office.
Colgan, F., Hunter, C. and McKearney, A. (2014) *'Staying Alive': The impact of 'austerity cuts' on the LGBT Voluntary and Community Sector (VCS) in England and Wales.* London: Trade Union Council.
Crawford, R., Cribb, J. and Sibieta, L. (2013) *The IFS Green Budget 2013, Chapter 6: Public spending and pay.* London: Institute for Fiscal Studies:
Davies, M., Porter, H. and Mitchell, M. (2016) *Implications of Reductions to Public Spending for LGB and T People.* London: UNISON.
Flanders, S. (2013) 'A UK austerity surprise'. Available at www.bbc.co.uk/news/business-23424527 (accessed 15 November 2013).
Hastings, A., Bailey N., Bramley, B. and Gannon, M. (2015) *The Cost of the Cuts: The impact on local government and poorer communities.* Available at www.jrf.org.uk/sites/default/files/jrf/migrated/files/CostofCuts-Full.pdf (accessed 10 July 2017).
Hunter, J., Cox, E. and Round, A. (2016) *Too Small to Fail: How small and medium-sized charities are adapting to changes and challenges.* Manchester: IPPR, North.
Knocker, S., Maxwell, N., Phillips, M. and Halls, S. (2012) 'Opening doors and opening minds', in Sutherland, M., Rivers, I. and Ward, R. (eds), *Lesbian, Gay, Bisexual and Transgender Ageing: Providing effective support through biographical practice.* London; Philadelphia, PA: Jessica Kingsley, pp. 150–164.
McNaughton-Nicholls, C., Mitchell, M., Brown, A., Rahim, N., Drever, E. and Lloyd, C. (2010) *Evaluation of Gender Equality and Equal Opportunities within ESF.* London: European Social Fund Division/Department of Work and Pensions.
Mitchell, M., Beninger, K., Rahim, N. and Arthur, S. (2013) *Implications of Austerity for LGBT People and Services.* London: UNISON.

Mitchell, M., Howarth, C., Kotecha, M. and Creegan, C. (2009) *Sexual Orientation Research Review 2008*. Manchester: Equality and Human Rights Commission.

Public and Commercial Services Union (2012) *Impact of Spending Cuts on Public and Local Services, Charities and Organisations for LGBT People*. Available at www.pcs.org.uk/download.cfm?docid=ED1C412F-EDD9-49DE... (accessed 19 September 2016).

Ritchie, J., Lewis, J., McNaughton-Nicholls, C. and Ormston, R. (2013) *Qualitative Research Practice: A guide for social science researchers and students*. London: Sage.

13 (Not) putting policy into practice

LGBT* ageing research, knowledge exchange and citizenship in times of austerity

Andrew King

Introduction

In the previous chapter of this book, Mitchell and colleagues gave a detailed overview of the effects of economic austerity on services used by older
LGBT*[1] people. This chapter[2] extends this by focusing on how my attempts
to put the outcomes and recommendations of a project I conducted on
LGBT* ageing in the UK into both policy and practice were shaped by the
same social, political and economic climate that Mitchell and colleagues
identify, albeit on a smaller scale and in specific ways. This chapter discusses
a project called 'Putting Policy into Practice' (PPiP), conducted in the UK
between October 2010 and November 2011, which was funded by the Economic and Social Research Council (ESRC) and undertaken in collaboration with a local government authority (LGA). PPiP was guided by concerns
about knowledge exchange and research impact; to ensure that, in this case,
LGBT* ageing research and the recommendations developed from it would
have an effect on the experiences of older LGBT* service users. The chapter will therefore discuss the methodology and findings of the PPiP project
in detail before reflecting on the significance of austerity for the project.
In so doing, the chapter addresses issues of emotional labour and LGBT*
citizenship, arguing that undertaking impactful research with and for older
LGBT* people in times of austerity has a number of 'costs', not least the effects on older LGBT* people's ability to be full citizens in ways that are un-
problematic for their heterosexual and cisgender peers. Overall, the chapter
argues that despite attempts by those researching LGBT* ageing to create
changes in policy and practice, we cannot ignore wider economic and political factors and how they interact with attempts to improve services for older
LGBT* people.

Attempting to put research into policy and practice

In 2007 I was commissioned, along with a colleague, to undertake a small
scoping study for a UK local government authority (LGA) to examine the

lives of older LGBT* people who lived and/or worked in the LGA area. The LGA covered an area that was very diverse, with pockets of both consider-able wealth and poverty. In addition, it was a very ethnically diverse area and there had been tensions between different ethnic, cultural and indeed LGBT* groups. Following the creation of separate strands as part of the reorganisation of equality and diversity policies in the 2000s (Monro, 2006), the LGA was at a point where it was committed to reviewing how well it was currently meeting those strands. As well as commissioning research con-cerning race equality, gender equality and a wider review of equality around sexuality, the LGA wanted to commission a more specialist piece of re-search that explored the lives of LGBT* people over the age of 50. This was something that was both innovative and significant at the time – there had been few studies conducted about older LGBT* people by policy makers and organisations, let alone academics (exceptions include Opening Doors in Thanet, 2003; Heaphy et al., 2004; Cronin, 2006; Davies and River, 2006; River, 2008; Fenge et al., 2009).

The study consisted of interviews and focus groups with a total sample of 23 older lesbian, gay and bisexual participants, as well as a thorough review of the existing literature on LGBT* ageing. Since none of the sample who participated in the study self-identified as trans* a recommendation was made that a further study be conducted to focus specifically on older trans* people's lives in the LGA area. The findings of the study were dissem-inated to members of the LGA and also to its associated service providers at an end-of-project conference. However, it was clear that both I and some key officers at the LGA felt that a follow-on project was needed in order to embed the recommendations of the study into LGA policies, as well as the practices of service providers in the local area and beyond.

A follow-on project, 'Putting Policy into Practice' (PPiP), was devised and came at a significant time, since it coincided with the emergence and insti-tutionalisation of the knowledge exchange and impact agenda in academic social science (Bornmann, 2013; Kitagawa and Lightowler, 2013). The im-pact agenda is based on the idea that knowledge exchange is the dynamic flow of information between researchers and policy makers/practitioners and ultimately this should have a demonstrable effect on a community of end-users. PPiP was funded by the Economic and Social Research Council (ESRC) with the intention of influencing policy makers, upskilling practi-tioners and, ultimately, making an impact upon the service user experiences of older LGBT* people themselves.

The PPiP project was built around a series of stages. Stage one of the project was an awareness-raising conference, which was attended by ap-proximately 70 people from a range of services, charities and LGBT* organ-isations. Stage two consisted of two knowledge exchange workshops with a smaller group of service providers and LGBT* community representatives and individuals. Finally, stage three was a final showcase conference which disseminated the project, including how it had been conducted, and some of the service providers involved in stage two of the project spoke about their experiences. In addition, speakers representing a number of LGBT* organisations gave their reactions to the project and discussed further work that needed to be undertaken. Ultimately, it was intended that the project would raise awareness about older LGBT* people and the issues they face later in life, encouraging service providers to shape their policies and practices with this group of service users in mind.

Each stage of PPiP had particular goals and outcomes. Stage one, the awareness-raising conference, was intended to encourage service providers to think about LGBT* ageing, to consider why the PPiP project was necessary and to enable those who attended to sign up for the next stage of the project. Those who attended the stage one conference included service providers, local policy makers, third-sector organisations, LGBT* organisations and older LGBT* people themselves. The conference included talks and guided discussions/activities. All attendees at the conference were sent information about PPiP and asked whether they were interested in taking part in the next stage of the project.

Stage two of PPiP involved the development of a workbook, called the SAFE Framework, which was used during the two knowledge exchange workshops. The SAFE Framework was designed to encourage service providers to ask themselves a series of questions about how their service impacted upon older LGBT* service users. At the first knowledge exchange workshop, service providers used this workbook to evaluate their understanding of LGBT* ageing and older people. They then had to create two action points that they felt they could undertake to try to make appropriate changes in their organisation or professional practice, with the needs of older LGBT* service users in mind. There was then an intervening period of approximately three months where the service providers tried to undertake these action points. They were also sent detailed information about LGBT* ageing and older LGBT* people to help contextualise and further their understanding. At the second, follow-up workshop, service providers reflected on the opportunities and challenges of putting their action points into practice and looked at ways in which they might be able to keep the momentum of their actions going once the project had finished, as well as provoke further change.

At stage three, the PPiP project was shared with a wider national audience at a showcase conference. A number of service providers who had taken part discussed their experiences, and there were other presentations about LGBT* ageing from academics, charities and organisations. At the end of each event, evaluation questionnaires were distributed to participants to assess their knowledge of LGBT* ageing issues in order to try to capture the impact of that event upon those present. Indeed, these questionnaires demonstrated that participants felt that the influence of the PPiP project, as a whole, would be primarily in terms of changing policy, but it also had the potential to change practices. In qualitative comments to open questions on the questionnaires, people emphasised the importance of raising awareness of LGBT* ageing, providing focused initiatives for change and, most significantly, how events like those on the PPiP project enabled them to meet others who also wanted to engage in this form of institutional action (for a more detailed overview see King, 2015). Hence, the events provided space for the formation of an informal network of service providers and others who wanted to engage in changing services and policies for the benefit of older LGBT* service users.

Key findings

PPiP was not an empirical research project in the usual sense: capturing service providers' initiatives, experiences, reflections and concerns through workshop activities and questionnaires provided useful 'data' about the issues faced by those who sought to undertake equality work to improve services for older LGBT* people. A number of initiatives were developed by the service providers who participated, including: introducing the recording of clients' sexuality in a sheltered housing service; using the Age UK older LGBT* Health and Social Care checklist in a medical setting; discussing sexuality and gender identity with care home staff; ensuring that staff in a housing organisation had an awareness-raising session provided by Opening Doors London; running a training session for leisure service staff; and acting as the organisation's first LGBT* champion.

When they were asked to specify what the nature of impact had been, 75 per cent of those who answered the evaluation questionnaires submitted at stage three felt that knowledge gained during workshops would have a lasting legacy for the policy, practice and ideas of their organisation. They were also asked to specify areas where they felt the impact of the project would be in the future, and they suggested: policy (65%), practice (73%), economic, in terms of better, more effective services (50%) and ideas (58%). In short, participants rated impact in terms of changes in practice as most significant.

Roadblocks on the journey

Despite the enthusiasm and engagement from a range of individuals and organisations, the PPiP project did encounter problems putting research recommendations into practice and, ultimately, with the changes that it was able to create. It became clear, at an early stage of the project, that service providers who wanted to participate were not always able to do so. In addition, more structural 'roadblocks' to participation were encountered. Some providers who did participate expressed their concerns about acting as the LGBT* 'champion' within their organisation. As others have noted (Colgan and Wright, 2011; Colgan and McKearney, 2012), there is often an onus of responsibility on LGBT* employees to do LGBT* equality work – either because they are 'expected' to want to engage in this form of labour, or because they fear that if they do not 'volunteer', then such work will not be undertaken. I can still recall with clarity the experience of a lesbian service provider who explained that she really wanted to engage in the project, but her line manager was both dismissive of the changes she proposed and her own motivations for doing so. As I have argued elsewhere (King, 2015), this means that LGBT* employees engage in a form of 'emotional labour' (Hochschild, 1983). Indeed, I want to argue that what is at issue here is a form of *queer* emotional labour that posits LGBT* individuals into difficult employment situations, *queered* career trajectories and affective decisions, which heterosexual and cisgender colleagues do not have to manage, a point to which I will return later in this chapter.

Six months after PPiP finished, all service providers who had participated were sent follow-up surveys to explore whether the actions proposed by them during the project had resulted in any longer term changes that may benefit older LGBT* people. While the responses to this survey did indicate that there were some tangible effects, such as still using a LGBT* awareness checklist for new staff and running LGBT* cultural competency training workshops, it was also apparent from the responses that participants were less than optimistic and some felt that factors outside of their control were having a negative effect on the potential to improve services with older LGBT* in mind; this was especially the case with changes wrought in organisations as a result of austerity.

The austerity context and the politics of knowledge exchange

As Mitchell and colleagues make clear (Chapter 12 (this volume)), there is a growing body of evidence which suggests that the politically motivated imposition of austerity in the UK since 2010 has had dire effects on LGBT* communities. This includes older LGBT* people and the services they make use of in their everyday lives. Mitchell and colleagues point to the direct effects of austerity on services (e.g. closure of specialist services), but also to indirect effects in terms of how services for older LGBT* people are able to function in such an austere economic climate, as well as to what extent LGBT* equality is prioritised or side-lined. It was, I believe, the indirect consequences of austerity that very much shaped the progression and outcomes of PPiP and thus had a very different form of impact upon the project than those purely related to knowledge exchange and policy/practice change.

Shortly after PPiP commenced it emerged that participants, although enthusiastic, had to balance competing organisational roles and pressures in order to attend events. Initial responses to recruitment strategies indicated that some of those who had hoped to attend were unable to do so because of staffing resources at their place of work. It was suggested by some people who were interested in attending that there were no longer enough people to cover their job or that recent organisational restructuring, in terms of who covered what services, meant that newer members of staff could not be left alone for such long periods of time while more established staff attended PPiP events.

Other participants claimed that they had not been fully supported by their organisation and had attended during their own time; that is, they had either attended outside of their hours of employment or they had taken annual leave in order to attend. In addition, some participants were unable to attend the stage one or stage three events for the full day and so missed the afternoon impact-generating sessions. Thus, the ability of the project to make an impact and indeed to measure this was somewhat circumscribed by these organisational factors, particularly the need to maintain strained staffing levels.

While the above examples refer to soft, mostly anecdotal evidence, they should not be ignored, since they reflect organisational problems found in similar research: that LGBT* equality work is regarded as less important in a hierarchy of needs when compared to keeping front-line services staffed (McNulty et al., 2010). Indeed, as Monro (2010) has noted, since sexuality and indeed gender identity are viewed as 'private' issues, they are more prone to being marginalised. There is a danger of creating an equality hierarchy whereby those elements related to sexuality and/or gender identity become marginalised and the intersections among equality strands are downplayed.

It is difficult to ascertain the degree to which the aforementioned factors were exacerbated by austerity. Similar research conducted before austerity began to take effect suggests that LGBT* equality work is sometimes regarded in a cursory way, despite legal requirements to promote it (Monro, 2006). Although such initiatives are now regarded as obligatory by managers (Colgan and Wright, 2011), employees may see adherence to these initiatives as more equivocal, especially when front-line services are squeezed and cutbacks have to be made. Hence, austerity and the organisational restructuring it creates may reinforce existing barriers.

PPiP had aimed to bring both managers and front-line workers together; to address issues raised by other researchers about who drives organisational change (Colgan and Wright, 2011). However, the extent to which those who engaged in the stage two workshops were able to implement change in their organisation was highly variable. In a response to the six-month follow-up survey, one social care worker explained that while her line manager recognised the importance of improving their services for older LGBT* clients, actually taking practical steps, such as producing a set of guidelines for other members of staff, was proving difficult to enact. Competing pressures, including time constraints, but particularly financial resources, were intervening and lessening the impact of the actions she had hoped to put into practice.

Therefore, the question concerning where impact is most effectively generated remains contentious. Is it at the top, senior management, level, which then trickles down an organisation; or is it at a practitioner, grounded level which then creates the climate for wider organisational change (Monro, 2006; Colgan and Wright, 2011)? Again, austerity may impact upon these lines of action – if managers are under pressure to restructure services or are moved from job to job, actually enacting change may prove difficult. If front-line workers are similarly moved around, or forced to cover more and more jobs, the opportunities for engaging in detailed, painstaking LGBT* equality work may be lessened, since it needs time and resources to embed and does not depend solely on the energies of individuals.

Like previous research, PPiP found that a significant amount of impact was dependent on goodwill and good communication among different groups/individuals within an organisation and the personalities and values of those involved (Richardson and Monro, 2013). Here again, these drivers may be adversely affected in times of austerity when organisational restructuring/redundancies can disrupt staff relationships and networks built over a period of time. Indeed, as Mitchell and colleagues (Chapter 12, this volume) report, restructuring is unlikely to be sustainable in the long term. In such a case, a cursory, 'tick-box' approach to equality work noted by others (Richardson and Monro, 2013) may be encouraged as more strategic, developmental work is fragmented and work that recognises the complexity and intersectionality of LGBT* experiences is overlooked.

Queering emotional labour

Given the importance of relationships to drive change in organisations and to promote better services for older LGBT* people, as I noted earlier, it is also important to consider the affective experiences of participants engaged in such work. There was much discussion in the PPiP workshops about developing, extending and supporting affective relationships with older LGBT* clients, not least that many of the service providers wanted to ensure a welcoming, friendly and above all emotionally inclusive service was going to be provided, i.e. not making older LGBT* people feel uncomfortable or distrustful. The concept of 'emotional labour' (Hochschild, 1983) has been much debated and applied to a whole range of employment situations and, indeed, to employees (Brook, 2009). It captures the way in which emotions are used in the labour process, in people's work and the effects this has on employees and customers/clients. Rumens (2011) has also drawn attention to the emotional attachments formed between colleagues of differing sexual orientations and the importance of this for individuals and the workplace more generally. My contention here is that many aspects of PPiP and the way in which services might be improved for older LGBT* people draw upon the affective experiences of LGBT* service providers and, in the case of PPiP itself, the older LGBT* advocates who participated in the project; a *queered* emotional labour.

During a stage two workshop, one participant, a service provider, explained that although glad to have participated, the project had generated a number of conflicting emotional responses for her. She was pleased to be undertaking something positive, improving her service for potential older LGBT* clients, but this also caused her some discomfort. She was acutely aware that other people within her organisation, particularly her line manager, dismissed the action points she was attempting to undertake because of her own sexual identity; in other words, while she fulfilled a role, being a lesbian who was 'out' to her colleagues meant that this was then reduced in importance as a consequence. The work she was trying to do was viewed as personal, as an emotive reaction, rather than as a professional role. Such experiences are reminiscent of those found in studies by Colgan and colleagues (Colgan et al., 2007, 2009; Colgan and McKearney, 2012) and others (Humphrey, 1999) who have highlighted how LGBT* employees are often compelled to negotiate personal and professional identities and how organisations, consequently, diminish their equality work. Here again, austerity may intersect and emphasise these issues. In responding to the six-month follow-up survey, one lesbian home care worker indicated that she had volunteered to be a LGBT* champion in her organisation because there were no resources for the role/work and it would not have happened otherwise. In this way, the services offered to older LGBT* people may be heavily reliant on the queer emotional labour of LGBT* employees and simultaneously 'downgraded' as a result. This is not to suggest that only non-LGBT* individuals should undertake such work; far from it. However, it does point to the need to reflexively consider the affective experience for LGBT* employees and the reactions of others to the work they undertake, especially in a climate of austerity.

There are also ramifications when considering the role of older LGBT* community members who participate in projects of this kind, or who undertake advocacy work in organisations in austere times. Some older LGBT* people who participated in PPiP clearly relished the opportunity to explain to service providers (of whatever gender identity and/or sexuality) how their needs were currently not being met; for them it was a cathartic experience and a form of giving back to their community. But others expressed a more tenuous involvement, feeling that they wanted to be involved in improving services, but aware that this took up time and energy. This variability has been commented on in previous participatory action research with older lesbian and gay people (Fenge et al., 2009; Fenge, 2010). Moreover, there is also a danger that certain voices are privileged in the process and others remain muted. In PiPP, very few of the older LGBT* people who participated were from ethnic minorities or from working-class groups. Others have suggested that volunteering among LGBT* people from these groups may be lower for cultural and/or economic reasons (Ward et al., 2008), and that this perpetuates the silencing and lack of ethnic diversity in LGBT* ageing research and policy provision, as noted by Westwood and colleagues (Chapter 7, this volume). Hence, knowledge exchange projects and wider LGBT* ageing equality work may privilege white, middle-class concerns and ideas about ageing among LGBT* people and further marginalise others.

There is, however, another aspect to this when viewed through the prism of austerity. Arguably, being impactful in times of limited funds requires the affective, economic and social resources of older LGBT* people whose sexual and gendered citizenship is then (re)appropriated, transformed and potentially turned into a commodification of self that is tied to a politics of development (Bell and Binnie, 2000). Or, as this could relate to older LGBT* people, to a discourse of active ageing that emphasises the importance of volunteering in later life (Walker, 2008) and implies that those who do not do this are somehow less community oriented and giving. By this I mean that the subjectivity of these volunteers is utilised to address institutional concerns and, as such, they are institutionalised, in particular ways, as a consequence. They are asked to represent 'Older LGBT* people' as if this is a monolithic community, rather than one that is multidimensional and intersectional, as a number of chapters in this book demonstrate. Hence, what may, inadvertently, be created by undertaking knowledge exchange work with LGBT* older people in times of austerity is a governing of self along institutionalised lines that may, at times, be at odds with what these older people want or require; they may be shaped as specific subjects in certain ways and not others. Therefore, those conducting this form of equality work must consider how it engages people as members of an older LGBT* community; although it can be positive, it may simultaneously be manipulative and occlude difference under the remit of diversity.

Constraining older LGBT* citizenship(s)

This brings me to a point in this discussion where I would like to explore the utility of the concept of sexual citizenship, which has become ubiquitous in discussions about LGBT* rights, policies and forms of inclusion and belonging in recent years, and to consider what this means more widely for older LGBT* people. Weeks (1998, 2010) suggests that the sexual citizen is a 'hybrid' being who represents and reflects wider social and historical transformations. The sexual citizen, according to Weeks, has new-found rights related to the sexual; and when discussing the rights of lesbian and gay people, in particular, Weeks suggests that sexual citizenship has come after a 'moment of transgression' (2010, p. 115). In essence, Weeks is arguing that transgression and inclusion are reflexive, continual processes, bolstering one another. He gives the example of same-sex marriage rights and suggests that this is both transgressive in that it challenges normative concepts of marriage as a heterosexual institution, but also inclusive in that it draws same-sex couples into the sphere of legal marriage. In effect, it is both transgressive and inclusive.

What Weeks provides with his formulation of sexual citizenship is, I think, a very useful way of considering rights claims and indeed forms of equality work that are being put into practice, as entities that are double-edged; something is gained, but it is always gained within certain conditions and parameters. Hence, rights gained pertaining to sexuality have shaped the lives and experiences of older LGBT* people; they have created freedoms, but these have come with constraints, as framing particular ways of living and being an LGBT* person.

It is a focus on conditionality and the shaping of sexual rights within normative frameworks that has concerned other writers in this field, particularly Diane Richardson (2000a, 2000b, 2004, 2017). While Richardson concurs with Weeks in viewing rights claims as central to sexual citizenship, she is more concerned about a second aspect, noting: 'we can conceptualize sexual citizenship in a much broader sense in terms of access to rights more generally. In other words, how are various forms of citizenship status dependent upon a person's sexuality?' (Richardson, 2000b, p. 107). Where Weeks rightly emphasises the ebb and flow of agency, the extent to which individuals can act and change their social circumstances, Richardson focuses on the containment of sexual rights within heterosexual frameworks; for instance, how lesbian, gay and bisexual people's rights are given in accordance with normative heterosexuality, rather than how they disrupt it.

Sexual citizenship, as a concept, is not without criticism, including revision and reconsideration by some of the instigators of the concept itself (for an excellent overview and critical discussion see Richardson, 2017). Indeed, for those of us concerned with LGBT* ageing, the notion of sexual citizenship has not always paid sufficient attention to changes across the life course (King, 2016), nor to issues around gender identity and trans*. Indeed, Pearce (Chapter 5, this volume) cogently explains why trans* individuals may experience a queering of the life course that can disrupt access to and inclusion within a whole range of rights and temporal-spatial locations. For this reason, I think it is perhaps more useful to talk here about LGBT* citizenship and ageing: the rights, sense of belonging and identity, as well as issues of inclusion and exclusion that affect LGBT* people across the life course, in different ways, at different points in time and place, and how these accumulate and create divisions later in life. Moreover, I think it is important to consider how LGBT* citizenship, as it relates to LGBT* ageing, is shaped and constrained by issues of austerity identified in this chapter thus far.

The rights of older LGBT* people will be curtailed if services do not recognise them, support and encourage their social networks, prevent stigmatisation and prejudice and act swiftly if harassment or hate crime occurs. This effectively means it is imperative that there is a focus on two fundamental problems: first, older LGBT* people's citizenship is curtailed when policy makers are prevented from formulating policies that can be put into practice; second, that a foreshortened form of citizenship is potentially being (re)created that generates a binary division between LGBT* people and cis/hetero people later in life.

It is clear from the evidence presented earlier in this chapter, but also in the preceding chapter by Mitchell and colleagues that both of the problems I have identified are in process. Austerity and the climate of cutbacks, closures and subsequent restructurings are having effects on policies and practices that need to be developed to ensure that older LGBT* citizens have access to equality in services and that they are not disadvantaged when compared to their heterosexual and cisgender peers. If a policy to further equality for older LGBT* people cannot be put into practice because the economic and political climate makes it impossible, then that climate is discriminatory.

Conclusion

In this chapter I have outlined a project which sought to take the findings of research concerning LGBT* ageing and the recommendations developed from it and put them into practice. The chapter has discussed at length how a methodology of knowledge exchange was developed and deployed in order to try to achieve this aim. Thus, the chapter has shown how a specific project sought to have an impact upon the lives of older LGBT* service users. However, the chapter has also examined how the socio-economic and political climate of austerity shaped the possibilities and potentialities of this project; to an extent, I have argued that austerity curtailed the ability to put research and policy into practice. When researchers talk about impact they nearly always focus on how to achieve it, what methods may be used and what positive outcomes may result. In this chapter, I have concentrated on the wider contextual barriers to impact, and the negative impacts of the wider context at a more micro-level. The chapter has argued that as a consequence the queer emotional labour of individuals is used in such a climate in certain ways, which may or may not be somewhat exploitative. By this I do not mean that taking part in equality work for older LGBT* exploits individuals per se, but it has the potential, when conducted under a climate of austerity, to be manipulative in terms of how their affective responses and labour are deployed and to what ends. Towards the end of the chapter I also introduced the notion of LGBT* citizenship, taking inspiration from the works of Jeffrey Weeks and Diane Richardson. The point in doing this was to illustrate and conceptualise how austerity can impact upon the citizenship of older LGBT* people. Austerity impacts upon the ways in which older LGBT* people do, or do not as I think is more the case, receive equality as they should under the law in the services that they engage with later in life. Certainly more research is needed to investigate this and my claims here are more conceptual in nature than fully empirically grounded. Nonetheless, issues about belonging and inclusion are currently dominating UK society, and in such a climate I think that keeping a watchful and critical eye on austerity and its effects on older LGBT* people remains vital.

200 *Andrew King*

Notes

1 Trans* is an umbrella term which covers the gender identity spectrum: including (but not limited to) transgender, transsexual, transvestite, genderqueer, gender-fluid, non-binary, genderless, agender, non-gendered, third gender, two-spirit and bigender (Tompkins, 2014).
2 This chapter draws upon and extends work published in King (2015) and King (2016)

References

Bell, D. and Binnie, J. (2000) *The Sexual Citizen: Queer politics and beyond.* Oxford: Polity Press.

Bornmann, L. (2013) 'What is societal impact of research and how can it be assessed? A literature survey', *Journal of the American Society for Information Science and Technology,* 64(2): 217–233.

Brook, P. (2009) 'In critical defence of 'emotional labour': Refuting Bolton's critique of Hochschild's concept', *Work, Employment and Society,* 23(3): 531–548.

Colgan, F., Creegan, C., McKearney, A. et al. (2007) 'Equality and diversity policies and practices at work: Lesbian, gay and bisexual workers', *Equal Opportunities International,* 26(6): 590–609.

Colgan, F. and McKearney, A. (2012) 'Visibility and voice in organisations: Lesbian, gay, bisexual and transgendered employee networks', *Equality, Diversity and Inclusion: An International Journal,* 31(4): 359–378.

Colgan, F. and Wright, T. (2011) 'Lesbian, gay and bisexual equality in a modernizing public sector 1997–2010: Opportunities and threats', *Gender Work and Organization,* 18(5): 548–570.

Colgan, F., Wright, T., Creegan, C. et al. (2009) 'Equality and diversity in the public services: Moving forward on lesbian, gay and bisexual equality?', *Human Resource Management Journal,* 19(3): 280–301.

Cronin, A. (2006) 'Sexuality in gerontology: A heteronormative presence, a queer absence', in Daatland, SO. and Biggs, S. (eds), *Ageing and Diversity: Multiple pathways and cultural migrations.* Bristol: Policy Press, pp. 107–122.

Davies, P. and River, L. (2006) 'Being taken seriously: The Polari in Partnership project – Promoting change for older lesbians, gay men and bisexuals', London: Polari. Available online at www.casweb.org/polari/file-storage/> (accessed 31 October 2008).

Fenge, LA. (2010) 'Striving towards inclusive research: An example of participatory action research with older lesbians and gay men', *British Journal of Social Work,* 40(3): 878–894.

Fenge, LA., Fannin, A., Armstrong, A. et al. (2009) 'Lifting the lid on sexuality and ageing: The experiences of volunteer researchers', *Qualitative Social Work,* 8(4): 509–524.

Heaphy, B., Yip, AKT. and Thompson, D. (2004) 'Ageing in a non-heterosexual context', *Ageing and Society,* 24(6): 889–902.

Hochschild, AR. (1983) *The Managed Heart: The commercialization of human feeling.* Berkeley: University of California Press.

Humphrey, J. (1999) 'Organizing sexualities, organized inequalities: Lesbians and gay men in public service occupations', *Gender, Work and Organization,* 6(3): 134–151.

King, A. (2015) 'Prepare for impact? Reflecting on knowledge exchange work to improve services for older LGBT people in times of austerity', *Social Policy and Society,* 14(1): 15–27.

King, A. (2016) *Older Lesbian, Gay and Bisexual Adults: Identities, intersections and institutions.* London: Routledge.

Kitagawa, F. and Lightowler, C. (2013) 'Knowledge exchange: A comparison of policies, strategies, and funding incentives in English and Scottish higher education', *Research Evaluation,* 22(1): 1–14.

McNulty, A., Richardson, D. and Monro, S. (2010) 'Lesbian, gay, bisexual and trans (LGBT) equalities and local governance: Research report for practitioners and policy makers'. Newcastle: Newcastle University. Available athttp://research.ncl. ac.uk/selg/documents/selgreportmarch2010.pdf (accessed 26 June 2013).

Monro, S. (2006) 'Evaluating local government equalities work: The case of sexualities initiatives in the UK', *Local Government Studies,* 32(1): 19–39.

Monro, S. (2010) 'Sexuality, space and intersectionality: The case of lesbian, gay and bisexual equalities initiatives in UK local government', *Sociology,* 44(5): 996–1010.

Opening Doors in Thanet. (2003) 'Equally different: Report on the situation of older lesbian, gay, bisexual and transgendered people in Thanet, Kent', available at www.casweb.org/polari/file-storage/index?folder_id=34791&n_past_days=99999> (accessed 31 October 2008).

Richardson, D. (2000a) 'Claiming citizenship? Sexuality, citizenship and lesbian/ feminist theory', *Sexualities,* 3(2): 255–272.

Richardson, D. (2000b) 'Constructing sexual citizenship', *Critical Social Policy,* 20(1): 105–135.

Richardson, D. (2004) 'Locating sexualities: From here to normality', *Sexualities,* 9(4): 391–411.

Richardson, D. (2017) 'Rethinking sexual citizenship', *Sociology,* 51(2): 208–224.

Richardson, D. and Monro, S. (2013) 'Public duty and private prejudice: Sexualities equalities and local government', *Sociological Review,* 61(1): 131–152.

River, L. (2008) 'Recent research from Polari on the health needs of older lesbians, gay men, bisexuals and trans people', *Housing, Health and Social Care Issues Affecting Older Lesbian, Gay and Bisexual People,* International Longevity Centre – UK, 18 November.

Rumens, N. (2011) *Queer Company: The role and meaning of friendship in gay men's work lives.* Farnham: Ashgate.

Walker, A. (2008) 'Commentary: The emergence and application of active aging in Europe', *Journal of Aging & Social Policy,* 21(1): 75–93.

Ward, R., River, L. and Fenge, LA. (2008) 'Neither silent nor invisible: A comparison of two participative projects involving older lesbians and gay men in the United Kingdom', *Journal of Gay & Lesbian Social Services,* 20(1–2): 147–165.

Weeks, J. (1998) 'The sexual citizen', *Theory, Culture and Society,* 15(3): 35–52.

Weeks, J. (2010) *Sexuality.* London: Routledge.

14 Conclusion

Minding the knowledge gaps?

Andrew King, Kathryn Almack, Yiu-Tung Suen and Sue Westwood

Introduction

In this final chapter we return to the beginning – the roll-out of the MTKG project – to discuss and critically reflect on our objectives, what we achieved, and we conclude with some brief thoughts for future research and practice. This project, which was funded by the Economic and Social Research Council UK, took the form of a series of six seminars/workshops and a final showcase conference (2013–2015). The topic of each seminar/workshop focused on a knowledge gap in our understanding of LGBT ageing: older bisexual lives; trans ageing; intergenerational issues and LGBT people; intersections of ethnicity, culture and religion; economics and austerity; and health, housing and social care towards the end of life. As we explained in Chapter 1, these six knowledge gap topics have formed the basis of the substantive chapters of this book thus far. In this chapter we want to discuss in more detail what took place during the seminars/workshops and the final conference, the knowledge generated at each event and what participants at the events saw as ways of taking that knowledge forward. Finally, we critically reflect on the process of generating knowledge in this way and discuss continuing gaps in knowledge about LGBT ageing and older people.

Minding the knowledge gaps

A central objective of the MTKG project was to bring academics across all stages of the career trajectory together with policy makers, service providers, third sector organisations, LGBT activists and advocacy groups and older LGBT people themselves; and to provide a forum for discussing each knowledge gap and thinking through ways to address it. Each seminar followed a specific format to maximise dialogue and generate new ideas. The seminars were day-long events and began with two speakers – specialists in the particular topic under discussion – addressing the set theme. This acted to outline current research on each theme and to identify knowledge gaps. Moreover, the presentations were followed by questions and general discussion, and these proved to be lively exchanges and reflected some of the diversity encapsulated in the audience. Although the presentations and debates weren't video or audio recorded, as organisers we tried to capture the essence of the debates in notes.

After a lunch break, a workshop consisting of small-group exercises then led into a feedback and whole-group discussion. The exercises usually took the form of a specific activity or series of questions to consider – participants captured their responses on poster paper and then gave feedback to the whole group. Event participants were also encouraged to create individual 'action points', things they intended to attempt to do in a personal or professional capacity to address the issues discussed, and again these were captured for recording by us via post-it notes which participants left behind at the end of the day. We also asked participants to complete an evaluation sheet at the end to assess the extent to which they felt the day had been successful in generating new knowledge and ideas about that specific aspect of LGBT ageing.

The project concluded with a final showcase conference, attended by over 100 people, held in London in January 2015. Baroness Liz Barker and Peter Tatchell were keynote speakers, reflecting on broad social and legal changes that have affected the lives of older LGBT people in the UK and what still needs to be achieved. Representatives of each of the six seminars/ workshops then summarised what had taken place and the knowledge generated at their respective event, and future steps were considered at a 'Question Time'-type panel. The afternoon of the conference was dedicated to smaller group activities, similar in design to those used during each seminar, and participants were again asked to complete an evaluation form at the end of the day.

MTKG events

Seminar 1: Older bisexual lives

The event was chaired by Kathryn Almack and held at the University of Nottingham on 24 April 2013. Two speakers gave presentations in the morning session: Sue George and Rebecca Jones. The afternoon workshop consisted of facilitated small-group discussions based on talking about case studies, to discuss gaps in knowledge about bisexual ageing.

This seminar explored gaps in knowledge about bisexual ageing, and how to address those gaps. Sue George considered changes in personal and social landscapes since her book *Women and Bisexuality* had been published in 1993. Sue also spoke about bisexual invisibility for those in same-gender (assumed to be lesbian or gay) and different-gender (assumed to be heterosexual) relationships. Rebecca Jones highlighted the many things not yet known about older bisexual people, and the importance of making work with older LGBT people more bi-inclusive. After a performance by singer/

songwriter 'Single Bass', the afternoon session explored older bisexual people's invisibility using case studies.

Key issues that emerged were:

- Identity: What does 'bisexual' and/or 'ageing bisexual' mean? There are different takes on this from social constructionist and essentialist perspectives. There are also distinctions between bisexual feelings, behaviours and identities; especially as these are seen through various cultural encodings and life course perspectives.
- Demographics: How many bisexuals are there and what is their distribution across ages, family types and other intersecting statuses? To what extent is bisexuality linked with key outcomes such as material, physical and mental well-being?
- Marginalisation: Several types of marginalisation, including within academic disciplines, within and across sexual minorities, and within and across age cohorts. Vastly under-represented in 'Older LGBT' literature. Prejudice, stereotyping and discrimination within the 'LGBT community' and mainstream society.
- Intersections: To what extent can research into the lives of older bisexuals address core issues in existing literature? Also, how is age relevant to sexuality more generally, and vice versa? Is there any material difference in the lived experiences of ageing bisexuals as compared to other sexual minorities and/or other generations?
- Access: How to do research on ageing bisexuals in the UK? How might researchers find them and to what extent does this limit the kinds of evidentiary bases upon which hinge robust analyses and the evaluation of extant or new theories in the social sciences?
- Lack of visibility: A combination of issues of identity, marginalisation, intersections and access issues in research.

In terms of ways forward, the following were identified:

- More research with and about older bisexual people.
- More research with and about older bisexual and trans people, who may share issues under the 'LGBT' umbrella.
- Greater visibility of and for older bisexual people (e.g. support groups for older bisexual people).

Seminar 2: Intergenerational issues and LGBT people

This event was held at the University of Oxford on 10 September 2013 and was chaired by Andrew King. The seminar began with presentations from Antony Smith, then Development Officer for Equalities and Human Rights, Age UK, and Catherine McNamara, Pro-Dean (Students), Royal Central School of Speech and Drama, London.

This seminar explored connections between older and younger LGBT people, the extent of existing links, how increased contact might be facilitated, and what the knowledge gaps are in this area. Antony Smith and Catherine McNamara presented their experiences in running three distinct LGBT intergenerational programmes, aimed at improving understandings and relationships between younger and older LGBT people and to develop knowledge and pride in LGBT heritage. The afternoon workshops involved discussions about future ways of improving intergenerational support among LGBT people and, working in small groups, participants were asked to devise possible intergenerational projects.

Key issues that emerged were:

- Informal networks: If LGBT intergenerational and multigenerational support systems were much stronger, it could reduce the need for formal care provision while reaping a huge social enrichment dividend.
- Social exclusion: Ageist exclusion within the LGBT 'community' as well as LGBT exclusion in ageing 'communities'. Possible differentiation by gender: older lesbians and bisexual women may have stronger intergenerational networks of support than older gay and bisexual men, especially as they are also more likely to have children and grandchildren; older trans individuals who transition in later life may be rejected by their children/grandchildren.
- Limited intergenerational bonds between LGBT people: Denies informal practical support to older LGBT people and also denies younger LGBT people positive role models, mentoring and advice.
- Need: To establish meaningful intergenerational LGBT relationships.

In terms of ways forward, the following were identified:

- More LGBT intergenerational research.
- Explore ways in which older and younger LGBT could offer reciprocal support.
- Practical solutions (e.g. shared housing; mentoring/befriending schemes).
- More intergenerational projects. Ideas included 'Connecting LGBT Generations' and 'Screening in, Screening Out' film projects; 'Care Share', an intergenerational time bank; and a virtual LGBT intergenerational community with shared online biographies.
- Making LGBT 'community' more age aware and ageing inclusive.
- Making ageing 'community' more LGBT aware and LGBT inclusive.

Seminar 3: Intersections of ethnicity, culture and religion

This event was held at the University of Nottingham on 23 January 2014. The speakers were Roshan Das Nair, Joanne McCarthy and Andrew Yip.

The seminar addressed the intersecting influences of race, ethnicity and religion in LGBT people's lives that have been relatively little discussed. Research has suggested that in addition to prevailing ageism, experiences of racism are not uncommon in the LGBT community. At the same time, LGBT people from BAME communities may also feel excluded from their own racial or ethnic communities that place a strong emphasis on family ideals and gender norms. Likewise, certain dogmatic interpretations of religious texts marginalise LGBT people from religious communities. In addition to such social isolation, racial discrimination throughout the life course can affect education attainment and employment market participation, which may also mean that some older BAME LGBT people may be financially disadvantaged in later life, resulting in barriers to accessing health services.

Roshan Das Nair and Joanne McCarthy spoke about their respective research that has examined the layers and levels of intersectionality of religion, culture and ethnicity, and the need to understand LGBT ageing as a complex, multidimensional experience. Andrew Yip addressed issues around ageing, religion and spirituality, noting the benefits, challenges and problems that they bring for older LGBT people.

The afternoon workshops looked at ways of increasing BAME inclusion in LGBT ageing research and activism, and the role of religion and spirituality in the lives of older LGBT people.

Key themes that emerged were:

- Intersectionality: Older LGBT people from BAME communities are positioned at the intersection of multiple points of discrimination. Often LGBT research and advocacy fails to address that issue.
- The need to consider multiple sites of social exclusion.
- How religion can be both a site of exclusion and/or support, and ways of changing that.
- Absence of BAME voices from LGBT discourse generally and LGBT ageing discourse more specifically.

In terms of ways forward, the following were identified:

- Develop work to address the under-representation of LGBT BAME staff and 'customers' in care homes.
- Work needed to reconcile 'fact' and interpretations of religious texts.
- More appreciation of the spirituality of older LGBT people.
- Much work to do to address racism in UK LGBT communities.
- Better understanding needed of the different experiences within intersections of race, age, sexuality.
- Importance of redressing gender/racial/age inequalities within the LGBT community.

- Where are older BAME LGBT people to be found in the UK and what are their (different) experiences? The most invisible/silent within LGBT communities.
- Creating dialogues across differences.

Seminar 4: Counting the costs? Resources, austerity and older LGBT people

The event was held at the University of Surrey on 29 April 2014 and was chaired by Andrew King. The two speakers were: S.C. Noah Uhrig, then at the Institute for Social and Economic Research, University of Essex, and Martin Mitchell, NatCen Social Research.

This seminar explored economic perspectives on LGBT ageing. Noah Uhrig and Martin Mitchell reported on their respective research projects to offer insights into the socio-economic circumstances of older LGBT people and the implications of austerity. Complex intersecting disadvantages were that those living in poverty are more likely to be affected by social welfare cuts during austerity. Discussions highlighted how socio-economic disadvantage needs to be analysed through the lens of both gender and sexuality.

Key issues that emerged were:

- Care and support: How can we develop appropriate care and support services for older LGBT people in the context of ongoing austerity?
- Social networks have both a material effect on older people's health and well-being and a preventive effect in terms of subsequently needing formal care and support. How do we nurture and develop those networks?
- Circles of disadvantage: Older LGBT people more likely to need formal care and support and to be affected by cuts to social care provision and/or loss of income experienced by charities during austerity. Lack of support from charities means greater need for provision from formal services, which are also restricted.
- Intergenerational relationships: If LGBT intergenerational and multi-generational support systems were much stronger, the need for formal care provision would be greatly diminished.
- Gender differences: Older lesbians affected by ageism and sexism, and economic consequences of gendered employment, gendered patterns of employment and the gender pay gap; gay men are particularly vulnerable to social isolation because of increased risk of living alone, ageist exclusion and less robust social networks.
- Need to understand more about economic circumstances of older bisexual and trans individuals.
- Socio-economic diversity: More affluent older LGBT people have greater choice and control over their formal housing and support options in later life, compared with less affluent older LGBT people, who have far less choice and control.

In terms of ways forward, the following were identified:

- LGBT community needs to embrace issues around poverty, austerity and social exclusion.
- Whether older LGBT people should be treated as a 'special needs' group, entitled to specialist funding, as in Australia.
- Whether this is a need for an organisation to represent the interests of older LGBT people.
- The need for more research which takes diversity among and between older LGBT people into consideration.

Seminar 5: Trans ageing

This event was held at St Thomas Conference Centre, Manchester, on 10 September 2014. It was chaired by Kathryn Almack. Morning presentations came from Louis Bailey, University of Hull, Ruth Rose, trans activist, and Jane McQueen, Press for Change and The TransEquality Project.

This seminar explored trans ageing issues. The morning speakers spoke about the range and diversity of trans ageing. The afternoon session was co-led and co-facilitated by Louis Bailey and Claire Jenkins, both trans activists. The seminar highlighted a wide range of issues and concerns for older trans people, and the need to address services and support, especially in later life. Recognising, respecting and validating diversity within the trans and LGBT communities was emphasised as a key issue.

Key issues that emerged were:

- Diversity among and between trans individuals: 'Trans' covers a spectrum of identities and/or lived experience; different issues for older trans women and older trans men; differences, for those who have transitioned, between those who transitioned early in life and those who have transitioned later in life.
- Depression: A major issue for (older) trans people, compounded by ageing.
- Frustration: Major problems accessing timely, appropriate medical support for individuals wanting to transition.
- Prejudice and discrimination: Opposition to continued pathologisation of trans individuals, especially those who wish to transition, and who need, in law, a psychiatric diagnosis in order to do so and/or to comply with the Gender Recognition Act.
- Marginalisation: Trans issues often conflated with LGB issues, including in relation to issues in older age.
- Celebration: Greater possibilities for later life fulfilment (and alleviation of depression) through increased opportunities to express one's true self.
- Concern: About formal health and social care providers being ill-equipped to recognise, understand and meet the needs of older trans people, especially in relation to personal care issues.

In terms of ways forward, the following were identified:

- More trans ageing research and more networking opportunities.
- Greater recognition, and understanding, of differences, as well as similarities, between LGB and T issues.
- More, and better, training for formal health, housing and social care providers.
- The need to continue to de-pathologise trans identities.
- Improving access to, and quality of, medical provision for those individuals who wish to transition.
- Need to address intersectionality among (older) trans people, including the needs and experience of trans individuals from BAME communities and trans people with disabilities.

Seminar 6: New directions in health, housing and social care: What do older LGBT people want?

The event took place at the University of Surrey on 26 November 2014 and was chaired by Andrew King. The two speakers were Kathryn Almack and Paul Willis, University of Bristol.

This seminar explored housing, health and social care provision for older LGBT people, and the associated concerns and preferences older LGBT people have about such provision. Kathryn Almack and Paul Willis presented their respective findings from recent research, highlighting the importance of raising awareness among service providers and developing a menu of choices of provision for older LGBT people, especially in relation to social and residential care and end-of-life care. The afternoon workshops involved discussions about preferences in provision as expressed by older LGBT people.

Key issues that emerged were:

- Sexuality often not acknowledged/taken into account in care settings in old age per se and LGBT expressions of sexuality may be doubly invisible.
- Older LGBT people may be invisible in a range of care settings.
- Recognising support networks which may be unorthodox.
- There was much debate about the pros and cons of LGBT-specific services/housing provision for older LGBT people.
- Need to recognise and work with both the commonalities and differences of LGBT experiences.
- Issues about eliciting 'sexual' stories, but perhaps older LGBT people don't want to discuss that?

In terms of ways forward, the following were identified:

- The need for implementation campaigns to put ideas into practice.
- Legal resources needed to set up a charitable housing trust and awareness raising around what is financially viable.

- More conferences to inspire discussion and policy change.
- Upskilling: Need help for activists to learn how to influence policy and common issues ongoing at local and national levels.

Final showcase conference

This large event took place at The Abbey Centre, Westminster, London, on 28 January 2015. The event was divided into a number of different sections. There were keynote presentations from Baroness Liz Barker and Peter Tatchell. A panel then had feedback from each of the seminars; these were: Sue George, author of *Women and Bisexuality*; Catherine McNamara, co-founder of Gendered Intelligence and Deputy Dean of Studies at Central School of Speech and Drama; Roshan das Nair, Consultant Clinical Psychologist, Nottingham University Hospitals; Kat Gupta, activist; Claire Jenkins, campaigner for trans and LGBT communities; Sue Westwood; and Paul Willis, Senior Lecturer in Social Work at Swansea University (now at Bristol University). There was also an 'Older LGBT – Question Time' panel with Antony Smith, then Age UK; James Taylor, then Stonewall; Jenny-Anne Bishop, campaigner for trans and LGBT communities; Rebecca Jones, Senior Lecturer, Open University; Vernal Scott, author of *God's Other Children*; and Tina Wathern, Stonewall Housing. There was also a poem reading by Sue Lister and a presentational talk by the writer, dramatist, singer-songwriter and comedian Clare Summerskill.

Over 100 people attended the conference. Towards the end of the day, those attending were asked to reflect on the conference and the MTKG project as a whole. The feedback on both was overwhelmingly positive, and included:

- "I really enjoyed the aspects of the seminars that have been based on the dissemination of research. Many of the speakers have been really well informed and have given excellent presentations."
- "I thought it was very good introduction for a range of issues and would lead well into further themed conferences."
- "Thanks for a welcoming and well-chaired event."
- "Very good to have info re: all the outcomes of the seminars – lot of work. Thank you."
- "This was a very useful event and a nice ending to the series."
- "This has been a very good day – buzzing with ideas and connections."
- "A great conference! Touched upon different factors, which give much food for thought."
- "This has been a great series – thanks for them. Please consider the next series soon!"

Participants particularly valued the opportunities to network and to share knowledge and experience:

- "This has been a wonderful series of events and I am so happy that further networks and community will come from this. Thank you so much to all the organisers; spaces like this make us all feel so much stronger as communities."
- "For me this series of seminars has really facilitated a research environment developing. Mainly because it has been done over two years. This has allowed relationships to develop, ideas to flourish, and debate to occur. I feel it has and will push the research agenda forward. Very well done. It has been fabulous."

Some critical reflections

The MTKG project aimed to address topics related to older LGBT people, which, at the time, were under-researched. As this chapter has demonstrated, the project began to address knowledge gaps in specific ways: through bringing different audiences together; through opening up debate; through encouraging new ideas about taking issues forward; and by bringing the authors in this book together to address the knowledge gaps that existed. As such, the MTKG project has achieved much. However, a chapter of this sort and indeed the project itself would be incomplete without a more critical reflection on both the project and its outcomes.

As a result of running the events, we believe we have learned the following points. First, there is a need to continually ensure that marginalised voices are included, as well as those of more vocal campaigners. For instance, we had a limited number of travel bursaries for each event to encourage participation from those who have fewer financial resources, and any future research and/or older LGBT events need to take this into consideration. However, marginalisation among older LGBT people takes many forms, not just financial; important knowledge gaps remain around older LGBT people with disabilities and people with complex mental health needs, for instance.

Second, we learned that there is a need to include individuals who identify beyond 'LGBT' categories, or as one participant put it on an evaluation feedback form: "There needs to be an awareness that terms/identities such as lesbian, gay, bisexual and trans are themselves culturally loaded terms, that are not neutral, and can therefore exclude some people." This may especially be the case for those older LGBT people who have lived with overt stigma and discrimination for much of their lives, or those whose social and/or cultural background leads them to reject such terms. It is vital, therefore, that the voices of these individuals are heard as well.

Third, more attention needs to be paid to intersectional issues, especially in relation to race/ethnicity, but also class, gender, dis/ability, heritage, religion, geographical location, language and citizenship status among others. While we believe that the MTKG project achieved some of this, to an extent, there is still much more research and activism needed. In so doing, we need to think carefully about who is doing the research/activism and how inclusive it is, or can be.

Finally, we need to consider the sustainability of initiatives such as the MTKG project and its outcomes. After the final showcase conference a group of us attempted to set up a UK older LGBT people's forum. While there was much enthusiasm, like many such initiatives it relied on goodwill, additional unpaid labour and time. Ultimately, we were unable to maintain the forum without ongoing funding. Similarly, this book, although adding to knowledge about LGBT ageing and older people comes at a cost, not only in terms of sale price but also the effort of a range of individuals to bring it to fruition. With increasing institutional pressures to produce publications that can be audited in research excellence exercises, we need to keep making the case for books such as this which bring authors together to produce new, collective knowledge.

At the end of the MTKG project we made the following recommendations, which we think are worth repeating here:

1   There is a need to better understand diversity and intersectionality in LGBT ageing.
2   Older LGBT lives, with all their diversity, should be included in mainstream ageing research as well as in LGBT research.
3   Issues of difference, privilege, advantage and disadvantage within and among older LGBT people need to be addressed. Research will continue to understand both the challenges that LGBT people face as well as the resilience they display.
4   Both ageing/older people's organisations and LGBT organisations need to better represent, and give voice to, the needs, issues and concerns of older LGBT people. There is a need for an organisation which represents the voices of older LGBT people, similar to that of SAGE in the USA.
5   The LGBT 'community' and LGBT activists need to share responsibility to address and support the needs of the older members of their communities.

Conclusion

We have used the final chapter of this book to give more details about the project from which it has emanated. In an era when LGBT people may still hesitate to disclose central aspects of their identity in all settings; where there is still discrimination, hate crime and stigma, the need to keep minding the gaps in our understanding of older LGBT lives remains as pertinent and vital as ever. Furthermore, this work is even more important in a climate where funding cuts and neoliberalism have had many negative impacts and, in some areas, disproportionate impacts upon LGBT communities.

Index

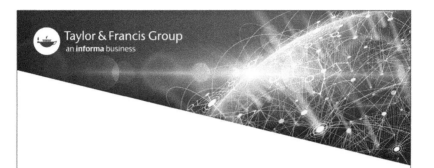

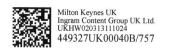

9 780367 586089